Last Chance

Last Chance

Lisa Keaton

To order additional copies of this book, contact:
Xlibris Corporation
1-888-795-4274
www.Xlibris.com
Orders@Xlibris.com
71453

Contents

To my daughter Haley.

If not for you, I wouldn't be here today.

Acknowledgments

I feel compelled to write this book in the years since the early 2000's when my body took a bizarre trauma that would forever change the normalcy of my life. This was the ultimate test for myself, my faith and my family.

First and foremost I would like to thank God for my miracle healing. I took on a journey that would only be in nightmares. I was transformed from a working class woman and mother of five children to a mere ninety six pound frame. I didn't ask for this, but deep down in my soul I never lost hope as I was launched on a downward spiral of grief and pain. I knew in my heart God assured me I would somehow make it.

My husband Philip whom was my caregiver, my physical therapist, my soul mate and my best friend. He saw me at my worst of times, and witnessed my first accomplishments. He had no doubt that God would heal me. Obviously with that kind of positive attitude, it made my life more bearable. I will love you forever.

I want to express humble gratitude to my children, Traci, Joshua, and Haley and my stepdaughters Sara and Katie. I especially hold my kids dear to my heart as they too suffered in their own way. Most of them were old enough to understand what was going on, but Haley at the tender age of two, something very wrong happened to her world and it came crashing down. She didn't know where her mommy went. This experience has brought her closer to me and she has blossomed into a beautiful young lady that is unashamed of being a Christian.

To my father and mother in-law Elton and Bettye Keaton for their unselfish support and love. They moved into our home and took over the responsibilities of parenthood which allowed Philip the freedom to stay with me. Even after I returned home, they continued to stay and help.

I express noble gratitude to the doctor's and staff at the Pearlman Cancer Center in Valdosta, Georgia and Shands Transplant Unit in Gainesville, Florida for their unrelenting devotion and dedication to their patient's care that pass though the transplant process. You are very professional and informative in your field. My case was very unique with challenges and struggles to overcome which at times were horrendous, but with God's grace, along with the bone marrow staff's "don't quit" attitude proved the most powerful experience of my life.

My "Daddy" Don and "Mama" Jackie Reuman of Ocala, Florida. Don and I went through our transplant together and formed an eternal bond. He was my father figure, my mentor and he never stopped encouraging me. I admire and love them dearly.

For my Pastor Mickey Wisehart of Faith Baptist Church in Valdosta, Georgia and my church family for all the prayers, cards, letters and support. Church's all over the country praying for my recovery and for that I will always be in debt, for you are truly gift's from God. I have deep gratitude for standing faithfully in our time of need. Bro. Wisehart, you would drive two hours to the hospital and sometimes wouldn't get to see me, but leave a card to let me know. Thank you for being a devoted pastor.

My most deepest love for my brothers and sisters and extended family who put aside their lives to support me during this unthinkable tragedy. Dale, you were Philip's right hand man and made the necessary medical decision's in Philip's absence. Philip seemed a superman on the outside and having someone close by also of a protective nature to understand where he was coming from. Someone to cool his frustration was more appreciated than you'll ever know.

Cousin's Jean Combs and Arbutus Guess who also served as caregiver and offered financial gift's. Jean, I learned how to give insulin shots without hurting you. I can't verbalize the love I have for you.

Particular thanks to Sharon Butcher and Valdosta State University staff for your gracious support of our family when I lost my job. I was the Assistant Manager of the Campus Post Office when I became ill. Sharon organized yard sales, a fundraiser and took donations in my honor. The University Alumni published an article about me and the national donor search to generate additional financial support. This was an unexpected blessing and much needed help for our traveling expenses. This was done cheerfully and has not been forgotten.

1

Even before the clock radio fills the early morning silence with music, Philip reaches over and turns the alarm off. He suffers from insomnia from years as a contractor. Going to bed with a deadline on his mind and schedules to prepare makes a restful night's sleep a childhood memory.

I turn over woken by his movements and see his wide-eyed face in the dimly lit room.

"I'm sorry" he whispers, now with his elbow propped on the bed.

"It's okay," I said sleepily, "I've got to get up anyway and take a shower."

While the other children are rushing through their morning rituals, I walk quietly into my daughter's room that is illuminated by a night-light which cast strange and grotesque shadows on the walls and her stuffed animals. I gaze down on one of God's most precious gift's to our family asleep in her little toddler bed. Her blankets twisted about like rope as she kicked them off in her sleep. I inhale the sweet smell of Jasmine shampoo and baby oil.

Haley is my youngest of five children and a true joy. At two years old, she is already a bright little girl who hints that she knows more than she lets on.

"Good morning punkin? How's my girl?" I half whisper.

She sat bolt upright, instantly wide awake, her face mixed with surprise and happiness. I bend down and pick her up, bottle, teddy, and all, and make our way to the kitchen where her brother Joshua and sister's Sara and Katie is busy preparing their morning meal. In no time all are fed, showered, dressed and on their way in different directions.

Philip leaves before anyone else, so I take Haley to the babysitter across town. Pat Best lives out of the way, but I don't quarrel about the extra travel time. I prefer the home environment with a motherly care giver. Pat is a large frame woman with a heart of pure gold. She once owned and operated a daycare, but since retired. She loved children and missed the interaction, so she made the decision to keep a few in her home for extra income.

I arrive at seven thirty and carry Haley along the neatly laid brick walk through the gate to the door and let myself in. The early morning air is brisk, so all that's exposed in the baby blanket is her nose.

"Good morning Nana's darling!"

Pat cries out as she reaches for Haley.

She had slept most of the eighteen miles over so now awake, a big grin radiates from her tiny face as she ducks her chin. Her look that says: "I'm being cute." Still clutching her empty bottle, she leans for the warm reception.

The pitter patter of other children scrambling around the room and the sweet smell of cinnamon rolls baking in the oven fills the air. One child hugs Pat around the knees to receive attention. I envied the children for Pat's unconditional love and home cooked meals. I softly kiss Haley one last time.

"Lub-ewe!" She squeaks softly.

"Mommy loves you too."

I could not even envision the chain of events that would take place that fateful day. February 24, 2001 would forever change my life.

After lunch, I return to Valdosta State University Campus Mail where I work as an assistant manager. After an hour or so I start to feel odd. That's the best way that I can describe it. My instincts tell me to not second guess my symptoms.

I am suffering from a vary rare form of leukemia called Hypereosiniphilia which caused great concern during my pregnancy with Haley.

In the early months of my pregnancy, my OB doctor found an unusually high white blood count, concerned she sent me to the Pearlman Cancer Center for additional test. From that point on I was under the cancer center's care. In my late thirties I was already a high risk patient, so this pregnancy was already off to a nail biting start. In the last trimester my condition worsened and on the sixteenth day of December I was admitted into South Geogia Medical Center Labor and Delivery for the induction to end the pregnancy. Haley Nicole Keaton was born at one o'clock the next morning. My daughter Traci cut the cord only after Philip was offered but he couldn't do it. Haley was handed to me with barley a whimper. I thanked God for this gorgeous gift as I counted ten fingers and toes. She was taken six weeks early, but a healthy five pounds. Haley was so petite that premie clothes engulfed her diminutive body. When she came home her Meme and sisters dressed her in baby doll outfits they had purchased at the local toy store.

I walk over to the manager's office. Sharon Butcher is very professional in her work ethic's which makes her seem snobbish to people that don't know her personal side. She likes to run a "tight shipped" office that reminds me of a school teacher I had in Elementary School. Mr. Newsom was the one that took on the task of paddling the student's which rendered *him* a fearful man. Most of the children preferred to stay away, but I knew the kinder side of him. My mother always taught us Davidson kids to "never judge a book by it's cover," and I always remember her words when I encounter a person different from myself.

I tap on the office door as peak inside.

"Sharon, do you have a second?"

Looking up from her computer and an unending pile of papers on her desk.

"Is everything okay?"

"I'm not sure. I think I need to go home."

I call Philip as I walk to my car. "I'm not feeling well, so I've taken the rest of the day off. Would you mind picking up Haley?"

Without hesitation, "sure, I'll call Pat and let her know I'll be a few minutes late."

Once home, I undress and climb in bed. Not sleeping steady is an aggravation as everything in my body ached. I felt as though I were catching the flu.

Evening came and everyone is home. Philip has all these helpers doing assigned task's that make a household run smoothly. He walks into our bedroom and sits down on the edge of the bed.

"Sweetie, are you still feeling bad?"

By this time, just a glimpse of him is comforting to say the least.

"I'm alright, really." I said with a grin.

"I just need to rest."

"Yeah, well, I'm going to feed the kids, and Haley ready for bed. If you're not looking any better when I come back in here, then I'm taking you to the hospital."

I didn't argue when he helps me get dressed. My body ached to the bone. The older children are watching over a sleeping Haley and settling down in their rooms themselves when we arrive at South Georgia Medical Center emergency room. Philip leaves me sitting in a chair and goes up to the window to check me in. After they are informed that I am a cancer patient, I am taken back right away.

Once in a room, the triage nurse ask the basic questions for treatment. After she leaves, Philip stands by my bed and begins small talk to pass the time. There is something about me that troubles him deeply. I am a strong willed woman that had accomplished an uphill battle since childhood. We are soul mates and he knows my thoughts, my worries, and my dreams.

The hardships of growing up in a large family without financial stability. The loss of my brother Chester at the age of ten while enjoying a summer day swimming in Lake Lanier. It was early in the afternoon when he fell off the raft and out of my life. My mother couldn't swim but made every effort to reach him. After five hours, at dusk the search was called off. As a rescue diver walked out of the lake, he stepped on him in the shallow murky water.

I felt for my mother's sake the EMT's performed CPR. My world fell apart at the seams as I stood on trembling limbs sobbing while I watched sand and pebbles pushed out of his lungs. It may have happened differently, but that is the picture I carry with me.

He was so little in his pale blue suit with visible scratches on his face and knuckles. He looked as though he was in a peaceful sleep in a tiny bed. Visions of my mother reaching in to pull him out and take him home haunt me. This was my first funeral. I was nine years old.

I have snap shots of my brother and I playing hide and seek around our house that was screened from the road by trees and shrubs. We listened to the wind whistling through the trees or the sound of rain pelting the tin awnings. We lived in an old house with large rooms and high ceilings. It's gray exterior gave it a forbidding appearance, but I loved the rambling pile.

My brother Dale took his death especially hard as he blamed himself for neglecting his younger brother. He was buried about a mile from our home in Flowery Branch Cemetery.

That was the worst summer of my childhood.

My brother Ray's tragic hit and run accident that took his life at nineteen. As he walked home from a friends house, he was plowed down by a man driving too fast. He was hit so hard it killed him instantly. The impact knocked him out of his shoes and his lifeless body was found in the brush fifteen feet off the road.

Ray had an irresistible smile and a way about him that made you want to follow him. He loved life and lived it wholly. He was a year younger than me, but he was the boss and I followed him. I remember one trip home from hiking in the woods. We encountered an electric fence. Angry at the obstacle, Ray urinated on the fence which gave him a nice shock. He could radiate the atmosphere with pure joy.

My baby brother Mike was killed one year later in an automobile accident, coming home from the same lake that Chet drowned in.

Mike, his twin sister Marie, and two other teenagers were in the cab of a truck. Several of their friends in the bed. The young inexperienced driver lost control in the soft dirt and the truck overturned. Mike was ejected and crushed by the weight of the vehicle. He died in the arms of his sister. He was sixteen years old. The youngest of the Davidson children and my mother's pet. She loved each of us in a special way but there was a particular love for him.

He had the enchanting ability to charm his way into anybody's heart. When I went home for a visit he would cuddle and play with my daughter Traci for hours on end. He loved to take charge in her care, feeding and changing her like a skilled father. He was buried next to Ray.

I lost my father several years later. A good man when he wasn't drinking, but a mean drunk. I sometimes wonder if he was elated when I arrived that early morning on December 3, 1960. The third child and first born daughter. Did my father express delight or downright disappointment for one more mouth to feed? To gain his attention, I was always a busy, tidy little girl, going around the house making sure everything was in its place. I had inherited his sparky strong-willed nature and qualities, but sometimes felt that I was a nuisance to have around. I craved cuddles and kisses from him. I remember very occasionally he would play card games or marbles with us on the front porch. That was a great treat.

I remember once he arrived home after work and saw me attempt with great difficulty try to ride my brother's bike. To my surprise he whisked me up in his arms and sat me down in his truck. I rode beside my father while he drove to the store to buy me a new girls banana bike. I was in awe of my father and prayed that he would stop drinking. I can still summon up the painful feeling of rejection, breach of trust, and isolation which crowd my memory. My childhood was very emotional.

My parents divorced after Chester's death and my father eventually settled in his hometown of Hazard, Kentucky. I never saw him again. He passed away from a massive heart attack when he was fifty six. He couldn't have suffered long, I hoped. With a massive heart attack he went down hard. Hard and fast.

He was buried on a hillside next to his parents in Red Hill Cemetery.

My mother was the matriarch and backbone of our family. She put her life on a shelf to raise her children and did whatever necessary to provide for us. She took the brunt of my dad's drunken rage to spare us.

At a very early age my mother instilled upon me the value of good manners, honesty, and accepting people for who they are. As I grew older, she told me that my life was, "going to be a winding road" and "dreams are just dreams if you don't work to make them happen." I remember how compassionate she was to someone's need, and taught us "to heal other people you have to suffer yourself." I longed for those days when I went home to visit and the smell of something appetizing baking in the kitchen. She succumbed to a twelve year battle with breast cancer and was laid to rest next to the boys. She was my hero and losing my mother has affected my life drastically.

I struggle to ignore my body aches without it showing. After half an hour of waiting Philip becomes agitated. White forms along his clenched knuckles as he paces the floor. He feels to much time has lapsed. Lingering at the curtain and asking anybody he encounters about the wait time.

"This night is busier than usual with all the beds taken and still more in the waiting room," a nurse explains.

"Please Philip, come sit down."

"I don't like to wait, especially when you're a special case here!"

Philip says through tight lips. His degree of protection for his family is instrumental and this instance proves no different, so to divert his attention I said,

"Look at that girl with cute toenail polish over there," gesturing across the room from us. A teenager dressed in a tennis outfit with an apparent injury to her ankle lay on the gurney. Her mother consoling her while holding a bag of ice on her foot.

"That color looks like something Sara would wear," Philip replies and we both giggle simultaneously. That's the last thing I remember . . .

2

Sometimes though, something goes wrong. A lot went terribly wrong that night in the small town of Valdosta, Georgia. He must have seen it coming. He opens his mouth to yell.

"Lisa!, Lisa!" Philip cries out as he leaps from the chair. *What in the world . . . . ?*

My eyes roll back and my body convulsing. While holding me, he helplessly looks toward the door. At that moment an ER doctor passes by the curtain. Philip sprints over and without explanation lifts the doctor up and around in my direction. Bolting into action, the doctor shouts for assistance. It is total chaos with all the nurses and machines moving in rapid succession trying to calm a tragic situation. The ER doctor directs orders to have Philip removed, but standing six foot five and two hundred forty five pounds that cast shadows over most average people, his insistence to stay is granted. Several shots of an antiepileptic drug is administered to halt the grand maul seizure. An IV is put in to continue the anti seizure medication. Philip's first thought, *she's not going to make it. Whatever caused this, it's killing her.*

"Mom, I'm here at the hospital and Lisa's had a seizure and they don't know why." Philip takes a deep breath in the attempt to control his jerky movements and continues, "she's been admitted and they're running a lot of tests. I can't leave her, so can ya'll come over and stay with the kids?"

"We're on our way!"

Philip's parents, Elton and Bettye Keaton live in Leesburg which is a little over an hour drive. Both retired so there are no restrictions or work schedules to resolve and arrive in lightning speed.

Philip follows the gurney to the X-ray lab for the MRI and CT scans. He is not allowed to touch or talk to me. Doctors have me deeply sedated and wants me to stay that way. My oncologist Dr. Eric Anderson is called and a constant report is given until he arrives at the hospital. After all the tests are concluded, Philip and Dr. Anderson are counseled on the cause of the seizure.

Pointing to the white specks on the CT scan, the specialist explains, "She has suffered twelve mini strokes throughout the brain, which caused the onset to the grand maul seizure. We won't know how extensive the damage the strokes generated until she regains consciousness."

After Philip leaves the room, Dr. Anderson is told that unfortunately the prognoses for recovery is grim and felt him to be the proper authority to further explain the situation on a more personal level.

Dr. Anderson speaks cautiously,

"I've contacted a neurologist to perform extensive tests on Lisa and we're going to do the best medially possible for her, but I want you to be aware of the obstacles she's facing."

With genuine concern of a doctor and friend he consoles Philip,

"I've always been honest with you and this time is no exception. If I have the slightest notion that she needs to be transported to a facility better equipped to handle this, you will be the first to know. This is bad, Philip. It's major. She is stable, but she's in a very delicate situation and her condition could change in a instant, so I just want you to be prepared. Okay?"

Philip fears that I might die without ever waking. With words hardly audible he asks,

"Should I call her family in Atlanta?"

Dr. Anderson looks at Philip obviously wounded,

"I think that would be a wise thing to do."

This is overwhelming, and he needs some time to himself; he needs some air. His chest constricting cutting off his air; he can't breath; his heart pounding so hard it takes control of his thoughts. Once outside in the Emergency Room parking lot, he falls to his knees and he prays aloud, "God, if you have to take one of us, don't let it be Lisa. Take me instead!"

Walking around the parking lot, he reflects on their relationship. He remembers the softness of her lips against his own. *Losing her would nearly kill me. Our marriage is still so young: where we are just beginning to discover the world together. Lisa has been blessed with the most tender of hearts, in many ways she's stronger than I am.* After several minutes, he calls my brother.

Dale is a retired Marine who lives on the family property in Flowery Branch. He works as a sales representative for a large hospital supply company, and his wife Marsha is a realtor. Their only son Scott is grown and on his own, which leaves them feeling isolated at times. Shortly after midnight the phone rings. With his best defense forward, Philip breaks the news to his brother in-law.

"I'll make arrangements and get there as soon as I can. Don't worry brother, everything's going to be alright." Dale assures Philip.

Marsha walks into the bedroom and looks at her husband packing his suitcase. She had been crying and through puffy eyes she notices that he had pulled out his dress suit he wore to the funeral home when our mother passed away.

"Oh no Dale, you can't take those!"

As the tears soaked her face. "Lisa's gonna make it, Dale, I just know it in my heart!"

He hugs her until the sobbing subsides and puts the suit back in the closet.

It is one of the longest three hour drive of his life. Memories crowd his mind of our childhood and how we were forced to mature beyond our years. His protective nature and father-figure persona kept the family together after our father walked out of our lives, leaving us to survive the best way we could. *Why now, why Lisa?* He thought.

While I'm sure the doctors did everything they could for me medically, I vaguely remember anything at all. I remain semi conscious of people working around me, talking to, and touching me.

Not until weeks later did I learn just how horrendous the incident was, and how close I came to not surviving it.

My first memory of consciousness is in ICU. I am oblivious of my surroundings and confused.

"Mrs. Keaton?" A nurse's voice breaks the silence.

"Do you know where you are?"

I open my mouth to talk, but I can't form words. All that comes out is slurred babbling. It is like my tongue is to big for my mouth. The sensation you feel after dental work and your mouth is numb. I blinked rapidly trying to clear my vision, but I see everything through smoked glass. I only make out shadows of people walking in front of me. I am not sure if somehow I have lost my sight or I am hallucinating. I thought I was still in the ER.

Within minutes Philip is holding my hand and talking to me.

"Lisa, something happened to you last night." He said as he wipes the droll off my chin. "Everything's going to be alright. I promise. I love you baby."

I turn in the direction of his voice and I mouthed to him, "I can't see."

Philip is a strong man and thought he could handle most anything. But here in ICU his fears are realized and he crumbles.

Shortly after my regaining consciousness, it is discovered that my left side is paralyzed; I am blind and speech impaired.

Swallowing hard, he prays silently for me to keep fighting, not knowing I am doing the same thing.

He talks to me constantly, keeping my fear at bay. It didn't take long for me to realize how profoundly my condition affected my emotions.

Soon, Dale arrives at the hospital. He and I are the two oldest Davidson children. We took on a lot of the responsibilities for our younger siblings. Dale enlisted into the Marine Corps to support the family and gave me his car so I could work and contribute also. During my mothers's last days of her life, Dale and I had to make the most difficult decisions concerning her hospice care.

"Hey sis," Dale softly speaks while caressing my forehead.

"I'd take this away and put it on myself if I could."

What once appeared relatively healthy and vibrant sister, now a hungry boniness to her figure. She looked frazzled after a long night of coming undone. Like a sick person willing to try any cure. Silently he greaves as he holds my hand for a long time. He always has a calming aura about him no matter what the situation.

Looking back to when I was seven years old, my mother allowed my sister and I to have a couple rabbits. They stayed outside in a cage built above the ground. One day, my rabbit got choked on some celery. Dale tried to dislodge it, but he was unsuccessful and the rabbit died. After consoling me, he placed it in a cardboard box lined with cotton, dug a hole by the shed beneath the old walnut tree, and laid it to rest. I'll never forgot that gesture of brotherly love.

A few hours later, my sisters make their entrance. My sisters and I believe in taking care of our own. They know me better than I know myself, so if I made expression that was a signal for action. Traci is the drill Sargent and squawks out commands for me.

"Is there anything I can do for you, mom?" she ask, and before I have a chance to reply, she asks something else.

"Is there anything I can getcha, maybe something to drink? Um, do you want me to get another pillow?"

All this chatter keeps my mind off my condition. Just having my family around makes my situation less stressful.

I silently make a promise to myself that now I have to think about myself for a change because if I don't get better, then I'm no good to anyone. This has opened my mind to the simple pleasures in life. I am taken aback by that person that lives in my mirror (who looks like my mother!) I would never trade my amazing family, my wonderful life, for all the riches in the world. My priorities have always been on someone else. I don't want to be here, but since I am, I have to become kinder to myself, and less critical, to become my own friend. I don't need to chide myself for eating that extra cookie, or for not making my bed, or for buying another cement lighthouse that I didn't need, but looks so avant-garde on my patio. I am entitled to a treat, to be messy, to be me. For heavens sake, I hope I get a second chance.

By late morning, Dr. Anderson's decision is made that as soon as possible, I would be transported via ambulance to Shands Hospital in Gainesville, Florida.

3

My deteriorating condition is a great concern for Dr. Anderson. The chances of survival are greatly increased at Shands. The hospital staff scrambles to finalize the paperwork for my departure while Pastor Wisehart and my family join hands around my bed to pray.

It is emotional. I can sense their pity, their sideward glances. How bad I had fallen.

I overhear the comforting words from a nurse say,

"I wish I was loved like that.

Pastor Mickey is truly a man of God and I have the utmost respect for him. He is a compassionate pastor who will often forfeit his plans to comfort a church member's need. He has spent many hours in a hospital or in someone's home, consoling and praying.

The EMT's put me on a gurney for transport. Our minister gives his contact information to Philip and speaks to me before leaving. My family escorts the gurney down the hall to the elevator.

"Sweetheart, I'll be waiting for you when you get off the ambulance. Okay?"

Philip says as he kisses my forehead.

"I love you," he whispers.

"Ready, Mrs. Keaton?" The EMT asks.

The ambulance is cold and drafty. This is the second time I'd been in an ambulance, but this time I'm in for a two hour ride. The EMT injects medication into my IV to help with motion sickness and in seconds I am drowsy.

There's constant activity around me. The EMT puts a blood pressure cuff on, hooks me up to a heart monitor and checks my IV line. His voice is soft and low as if he is humbled at the sight of me. He knows of my inability to see, so he informs me of his movements. I found him most charming and caring.

I am trying to stay focused, but as the drug enters my body, I become very relaxed. The warm blanket and the sound of the vehicle traveling down Interstate 75, my mind drifts to random thoughts of my life and children. Everything is crashing down around me, I have never felt such confusion, frustration, helplessness, and anxiety in my life. I can't get away from it; I can't make it go away. As I retain the memories of my children, I am constantly reminded of their need for me. I have so much to give: my walk in life can't be over already.

I see my children as if I am looking through a microscope. All together, yet each holding different memories. Seeing them as I had never seen them before. Traci is my first born and the apple of my eye. I was young when she came into my life and how I cherished her. She's strong-willed like myself and yet has a marvelous inner-directed laughter that radiates her charm. Her beautiful blonde hair and deepest blue eyes accent supernatural charisma. She has exceptional intelligence and a million-dollar smile. When she was young, I listened intently to her chatter holding on to every word. She became a second mother to her brother Joshua. When he was born, she had a real baby doll that she could dress up and carry around.

Fear engulfed me when I wondered if my vision would ever return to see her vibrate smile again.

My son Joshua comes into my mind. He has always been a mama's boy and I adore him. A tall, lanky sixteen year old and still outgrowing the gawkiness of adolescence. He has my ocean blue eyes. A cotton top for most of his life, now a dirty blonde. He plays all sports, but his first and favorite is motocross. At the tender age of four, this skinny little boy straddled a motorcycle and tormented himself for hours on end for a chance to place in a race. I worried over this brutal assault on his body and the pressures of competition. I remember on particular race, Traci and I witnessed him sailing over a patch of trees and crashing on a hillside. When we reached him, his helmet was covered with blood, but insisted on completing the race. He shouted, "please don't touch me or I'll be disqualified!"

The checkpoint judge did a quick assessment before permitting him to continue the race. Josh raced hard to gain ground and managed to place third. Later we found out he had a concussion and broken nose. He always puts his heart and soul in everything he does. He's my pride and joy.

Sara, my stepdaughter, is two years younger than Joshua and my golden child. When Haley called her "Sissy" at two years of age, that became her name. This title seems to suit her as she gives her love generously. Even as teenagers so often bestow an element of pride, she is a responsible young lady. Sara's the "taxi" for the family. If there is any errands or someone to pick up, Sara's called. "Sissy" is a package of unconditional love, hands down.

Katie is my youngest stepdaughter and a firecracker. She's special to me because she shares my mother's name. A brown haired long-legged, skinny girl with a boldness spirit. She has dreams of becoming a fashion model and although there is that degree of protection, her father and I support her.

The EMT breaks my slumber when I hear him shout to the driver,

"Oh man! Did you see that SUV?"

"Yeah, he must be in a hurry to pass us on the emergency lane!" the driver yells back.

It wasn't until days later did I learn that it was Philip, Dale and Traci that they were talking about.

I drift back to thoughts of my youngest daughter Haley. My pregnancy revealed I had an unusually high amount of white blood cells which later was diagnosed as this rare leukemia I'm now fighting. She is the reason for the discovery of my illness. I recall the day in the doctor's office, when she informed me that with my blood pressure elevated and white count exceeding ninety thousand, it was in their best judgment to have me admitted immediately and induce labor. I prayed that everything would be alright with the baby. Even though she was tiny at birth, she was otherwise healthy with no sign of the blood disorder.

Thinking about my children gave me renewed inner strength to fight this not for myself, but for them. I was going to do my best to beat this. God's now got my attention and I'm stronger in my faith than I've ever been. I'm learning that I can't fix this on my own; slowly, painfully, I am learning. I believed in my heart that God didn't want me to drag through life, barely making it. He didn't want me to be unhappy or to worry how I was going to take care of my children. I know this is not going to be easy, but if I set my mind to it and hold on to my faith, I will pull through this.

Sometimes when life doesn't go as I planed, or when I'm met with disappointments, I think, *Would someone else who has gone through what I have be able to except things the way they are. I know my doctor's have been able to keep me alive and they've done good things for me, but I'm so scared. When is this nightmare going to end?* The EMT touches my hand, "Mrs. Keaton, we're here. You're going to be okay."

The doors swing open, "Hey mama!" Traci yells.

It is a crisp February evening with a chilly breeze swirling around the entrance. I have no idea the journey my life is about to take, or how many setbacks I will suffer in my recovery. I am admitted to the medical floor for the first twenty four hours. Dale stays with me while Philip completes the necessary paperwork down stairs. My sisters arrive and wait with Traci for their turn to come in.

"She's checked in, so one at a time can come in to see her" a nurse says.

Traci is first.

"Mom, you okay?"

With a smile I nod. *I have to be strong. I can't let her sense my fear.*

Philip stands on the other side of the bed and says, "They want to do a procedure called leukopheresis. The process is like kidney dialysis and will filter the white cancer cells out of your blood. This will save your organs from any further damage. They want to start immediately."

He leaves momentarily to inform my sisters of the attempt to stall my deteriorating condition. There's a sense of hopelessness of the situation, despite of Shands doing everything possible.

It is extraordinarily emotional for my sisters to watch me go through the leukopheresis so Dale, Traci and Philip remain during the procedure. Dale stands with his hand jammed in his pockets while he watches me suffer. I am neither unconscious or medicated. I wish I was!

The medical staff are instructed to repeat the procedure a second time. As my blood travels through the filtering machine, cooling it in the process, and slowly lowering my body core temperature. My lips turn blue and I shiver uncontrollably. A nurse covers me with a hot air blanket, but I still shake like a leaf blowing on a windy day. The second leukopheresis treatment is successful and I am transported to a room.

"I'm glad that's over, sis", Dale says with a grin.

"I know this seems horrible, but believe me they had to do it go get you back on track. You're going to be just fine now, trust me."

I smile because I know my brother.

By now it's shift change, so everyone is ask to leave until after I am settled in my room. I feel at peace; I know I have survived a horrifying injury to my brain.

Hundreds of people are praying for me. I realize the miracle of prayer got me this far and I feel God's inner strength building me up. I will make a conscious decision to try my best to stay positive and do everything I can to help in my recovery. *I'm not the only one; I didn't ask for this, but God's chosen to keep me alive for a reason. I have to stay strong in my faith for myself, for my family.* Philip said earlier to me,

"I'll encourage and support you, but it's up to you to get well. If you depend on me, then you've accomplished nothing. Your drive must come from in here (pointing to his heart) not from me. You have to want to do it; you have to do it not for me or anyone else. Think how you feel this moment about yourself. Don't let that feeling fester into a mountain. Don't allow yourself to build on it. Take risks, keep taking risks."

Because of the limited space in the rooms, visitors are allowed a few minutes at a time and there are no pre-eminence in a case such as mine. A row of chairs lines the hall outside the unit and there my family stay until permission is granted to return. The male nurse instructs Philip to join my family in the hall beyond the double doors, so he doesn't have a chance to tell me that he isn't allowed back in my room until morning.

Incredibly my sight is returning, I'm able to see shapes of people walking in front of me. My speech barley recognizable I ask, "where's my husband?"

"He's not allowed back in until morning, so you can rest," replies the male nurse.

Embarrassed I ask, "I have to go, could you get a female nurse for me?"

"I'm your nurse tonight. I'll get a bed pan and help you in a few minutes," he replies.

As he is leaving, he stops and turns on the television to a sports channel.

"Do you like basketball? I love the game, but I can't play worth a hoot," he says and leaves the room.

I lay there waiting for him to return as the noise of the basketball game fills the room. My bladder is uncomfortably full. I blindly search all around and above my head for the call button. Frustrated I cry out for help, but my cries are drowned out by the noise of the television, and muffled by my weeping. I bite my tongue and my voice is raspy and raw. I have no voice left with which to shout. My pleas for help are reduced to whispers. Helpless and can't hold it any longer I let go and wet the bed. I am cold, soaked in urine and crying when the nurse walks in with the bed pan.

"What's the matter?" he ask, as he pulls back the sheet.

In an angry whisper he chastise me, "Look what you've done. You've caused me extra work!"

The next several minutes I endure his rude outburst and insults as he strips me and the bed naked. I can't believe this is happening to me. I sense his eyes squinting at me as he gathers the soiled linen.

"I'll be back," he growled.

I am humiliated beyond words. Left alone I feel helpless and terrified for the moment he returns. He has taken advantage of my inability to defend myself. *"I wonder how many patients he has treated like this?"*

As much as I fight it, depression floods in. I lay there naked and cold with no idea why this person is treating me this way. Adrenaline pumping through my veins, I am filled with panic while the nurse rolls me around like a rag doll. I can't find the words to tell him to stop. He is rough and indifferent towards me. I dare not challenge his authority. At this point I don't care: I am defeated and beaten down. I want him as far away from me as I can get him. I don't know how long I will be in this room, but as soon as I am somewhere safe, I will tell what happened tonight. He needs to be stopped. I wouldn't be able to point him out in a line up, but I know his voice. His every slur, every snarling derogatory comment that burns my soul. I will stay on guard for the rest of the night, not speaking or acknowledging his presence.

I find myself looking back to days long gone by, my brother and I walking along a gravel path leading from our house to a small pond off the beaten path. The North Georgia air was suffocating, and I am sticky wet with perspiration. The winding narrow trail was empty, as always. A cane pole propped up on my shoulder, I looked for the root that had caused my brothers bloody knee the day before. It took a moment for me to find it, at the base of a towering pine tree; protruded just under the dirt and across the path like a small snake stretching in the sun. the muddy water reflected our shadows standing on the bank. There was a faint odor of brine as I took my seat. I opened the coffee can of worms we had dug up in the yard and tore the first worm in half, the way Dale always did. Holding the cane pole tight I tossed the line into the water wondering if I would hear Dale add a few inches or pounds to the fish that got away that day.

After the morning shift change Philip is followed by the day shift nurse into my room. To his surprise, he finds me sitting up in bed.

"Lisa, how did you get up?"

"I wanna go home!" I cry, as I reach out and grab the sheet around me. "I feel like I'm in the "Twilight Zone". I don't want to be here. Take me home. Please take me home.

He holds me tight. "What's wrong? Please tell me?"

Philip and I have watched the Rod Sterling's television show "Twilight Zone" a lot, and he knew that I had to be in something very close to hell.

"I've called an orderly to transport you to another floor. You'll be leaving shortly, Mrs. Keaton." Says the nurse.

Once I am in my new room, Philip tucks the blanket under me, while my family gathers around the room. Philip can sense something is wrong, but contributes it to all the stress I've been through.

"Will I have different people taking care of me?"

Concerned Philip ask,

"Why are you worried about that, Lisa? What's wrong?"

He and Dale lean forward to listen. Promising not to take matters in their own hands, I tell them what happened while I was alone.

The call button is pushed and within a few minutes the hospital administrator takes a statement. I paint a picture of disbelief, humiliation and overwhelming sadness. She returns, apologizing again and assuring us of the nurse's dismissal and loss of license. There was a camera in the room, but obviously the nurse had turned it off.

"Abuse of any kind is not tolerated and is dealt to the highest degree. Shands is one of the Southeast's premier health facilities. Quality and patient safety are our top priorities. We are committed to providing exceptional patient care and service. Shands is dedicated to creating and maintaining a culture of service excellence. Our goal is to ensure expert medical care in the safest environment possible and our commitment is to provide you with the best care possible," said the hospital official.

I admired the hospital for their affectionate attitude and quick action. I am glad that I had come forward. This health facility provided excellent care for Philip's little cousin Jamie when she was a patient, I knew this was the place I felt most caring as well. I did not blame Shands for this incident. Maybe the nurse had private issues that wasn't detected by his peers. For this rapid action taken to remove the nurse and his license, I feel this was an isolated incident and if I need additional care in the future, I have no reservations about returning. I am elated that this man is forced to seek a different career field, so there will be no further cruelty to a patient. I don't hate him or hold a grudge towards him. If I can't find it in my heart to forgive him for his sin against me, then God can't forgive me of my sins. I'm afraid that people in this world don't listen to their heart, to often they are quick to anger and strike out. They let their feelings and emotions do the thinking. Sure people sometimes get on my nerves or aggravate me, but my days here on earth are too short to waste time over petty things. Anger and hate is like a deadly disease that can destroy a soul turning a person into a festering monster. It isn't easy to forgive but forgiveness will replace bitterness.

4

The twelve mini strokes affected the dominate side of my body. I am left handed, so my left side is paralyzed. The physical therapy is grueling, but necessary to regain motor control. It is difficult to explain to my children how I lost the ability to do things as easy as eating and walking that I learned as a child.

We are no strangers to Shands Hospital. Before my stay here, Philip's sixteen year old cousin Jamie Day was a patient. She fault diligently but lost the battle to a rare form of brain cancer more commonly diagnosed in adults. She was a beautiful young lady with a bright future and an inspiration to everyone. A playful sense of humor that could put anyone in a good mood; showing a tender and considerate and helpful nature. We were heartbroken with her passing.

I remember one summer in particular, we were invited to spend the day tubing on the Flint River with Philip's family. Joshua didn't want to go because he couldn't take one of his friends.

"Mom", he pouted, "Sara and Katie have each other to tube with and I'll have nobody."

"Space is limited on the boat, besides you'll have Jamie to tube with." I said.

But at eleven, boys are more comfortable having a great time with someone more like themselves. However, on our arrival, Josh was smitten at the first sight of Jamie and they became constant companions. She had that affect on everyone she met. At the end of the day, Josh and Jamie exchanged pictures and addresses. Joshua proudly displayed her picture to his friends. They remained close friends until her death. Joshua was a pallbearer at her funeral, so to keep from crying, he talked to her as he carried the casket.

Heaven gained another awesome soul that December day when she left this earth.

I have two therapists that work with me on alternating days. One works with my arm and hand, helping me with coordination and control, so the relearning process of eating and writing goes smoothly. The other therapist concentrates on my leg, keeping it flexible and strong for walking when I regain enough strength. I am determined to beat this and get my life back, or at least be able to go home.

"Considering what you've been through, we should have a great outcome." The therapist said.

On one occasion, I am given the task of feeding myself.

"You don't understand, she can barely raise her arm, much less feed herself." Philip explains.

"I'll help her. She's getting stronger everyday and we need to work on her coordination,"

He wraps my fingers around a foam-covered plastic spoon and with weak jerky moves I proceed to feed my eye, my forehead and my nose. I never make it to my mouth. The therapist is kind in his efforts to help guide my movements. After my session Philip leaves to get another dinner plate from the cafeteria.

For a woman who likes to be in control, this is profoundly disturbing for me to comprehend. The strokes have left me imprisoned in my body. My brain is like a filing cabinet turned over and files spilled on the floor. I can't think straight and very forgetful.

Philip is standing in the doorway even before I know he is there. How long, I couldn't tell. I look up and there his is smiling. He sits the tray down.

"Ready to feed yourself again?"

I roll my eyes heavenward. "Sounds exciting,"

This time he holds my hand in his and we practice the motions together. With his help, I fed myself. He happily submits my efforts to clean my face with a wet wipe.

I feel that he looks at me with new eyes, handling me like a precious piece of porcelain to be admired but not touched.

Next we practice my handwriting. I use an oversize preschool tablet with ABC's printed on lined paper. Philip mimics the therapist and puts a pencil into the rubber grip and wraps my fingers around it. I try to trace the letters. He's relentless in our private therapy sessions, careful to express only positive reinforcement, but in his heart, desperate to have me back. My efforts to write are in vain. The scribbles resemble toddlers art work.

"That's all right." Philip says softly. "We'll just chalk it up as a mile stone in your progress," then sets up a board game to play checkers. I strain to control my left hand to move the game pieces.

At times, he would sit and listen to my gripes and groans then when I'm done with my pity party, he explains his view.

"Lisa life is what you make of it. You can let what has happened to you ruin the rest of your life or let it be a learning tool."

"But I get tired and frustrated!" I interrupt. "I can't help but feel helpless. I can hardly do anything for myself, not even walk or use my hand properly. This is the most pitiful experience of my life. I'm like a toddler and everyone get's excited over the least amount of improvement. I never imagined myself lying in bed, half of my body unresponsive. I'm flat on my back most of the time, and the exertion to move takes extraordinarily effort. It's like a terrible nightmare and I can't wake up. I am a prisoner in my own body. I have empathy for those unfortunate people that have suffered strokes. Deep inside, I'm afraid that I'll be like this for the rest of my life. I feel that I've failed my children in ways to frequent to count, I can't help but wonder about life without me. I miss listening with interest whenever my children speak to me, and everything discussed seems new."

He continues, "You can't relive one second of the past. The damage is done and there's nowhere to go from here but up. Think about it, there's always someone else in worse shape than you, so thank God that you're alive and pray for him to give you strength to climb this mountain. I feel that God has a bright future in store for you and as you say, "everyday is a bonus day." Cherish this time, and let's work together to get you well, okay?"

"Okay."

Word spreads fast and cards and letters arrives in from all over. Pastor Wisehart makes several trips from Valdosta to deliver cards and gifts from our church.

"Lisa, you have prayer warriors from Florida up to Indiana praying for your recovery. This is a sign of people who love you," the pastor says.

I enjoy his visits and his uplifting praise and encouragement. At times I feel cheated until I catch a glimpse of myself in the mirror and feel guilty for being ungrateful of God's blessing.

In the moments alone, I pass the time looking down from my fourth floor window and watch the streetlights around the square popping on all at once, followed a moment later by the antique lamps along the sidewalk in the square. It is an appealing setting. All of Gainesville is like this; idyllic in many ways, safe and intimate and scenic, full of greenery and ponds and winding roads lined by century old oaks.

My memory tugs at me and a clip from my childhood springs up. It is my first memory of living in a rustic old school house in Hazard, Kentucky. It was probably among the oldest in town. Set back off the main road, dilapidated and abandoned for years until my father became the new owner. He labored long hours working as a coal minor, so evenings and weekends consumed his time renovating room by room until it was suitable for us to live in. He was meticulous in the work he did. He restored the heart pine floors that covered every room to their former glamor. My mother waxed the floors and we polished them to a shine by skating around in sock feet. I spent long summer days playing in the huge yard with thousands of wild flowers in full bloom. In the early evenings, my mother sat in a rocking chair on the porch embroidering doilies with the hope of catching a stray breeze. An occasional glance to check on my brothers and I walking in the ice-cold creek. A coffee can in hand poised ready to scoop up unsuspecting crawdads scattering from overturned rocks. A hearty laugh echoed from the porch when one of her children made a long, loud, piercing screech while jumping out of the creek with a lobster-like crustacean attached to their big toe. Even now, the old home place retains a look of grandeur that has only grown with the passage of time.

Philip's parents, Elton and Bettye, move into our home to keep some sort of normalcy for my children. Joshua moves to North Carolina where his father lives. Traci now married has a home of her own less than a mile away, so Sara, Katie and Haley are the only children at home. My kids are constantly on my mind as I work conscientiously on my rehabilitation.

I am a mother of five children, the wife of a caring husband and until all this, a woman with few worries. I was forty one years old, the picture of health and in good physical shape. Since my "brain incident" I knew I wouldn't be that vibrant, healthy woman again.

MRI's are scheduled at different stages of my recovery to evaluate my progress and brain function. Even though the reports are promising, I still feel skeptical of my abilities. Philip continues to help me with my writing, eating and walking exercises, most of the time not saying much. He didn't need to. His smile and tender touch is enough. *I'm so loved by my husband. I know it is hard for him—really hard.*

Everyday brought new hope, I fight my battle with superhuman will power. Philip walks beside me strapped to the walker. Five steps. Rest. Five steps. Rest. I feel like I could collapse at any moment, but I push myself to keep to my pattern. After all, I have a baby girl at home that I need to keep up with. Five steps. Rest. Five steps. Rest.

Over time my condition improves. I fight depression as much as I fight to get well. My security blanket came in the form of a six foot five inch husband. A gentle giant with gushing charm and bright smile.

At times, I own the world and other times I fall into the debts of pity. Philip is there for it all. He is able to calm a stressful situation and make it seem trivial. One day, I am extremely nauseated from a chemotherapy treatment and can't handle the hospital food, so he brings me a plain baked potato from the restaurant down stairs and it becomes my food of choice.

During my recovery period, I learned a lot about myself, about my faith. I don't like many things I can't change fast enough. I could at times just give up and be satisfied to live in peace without the pressure to constantly trying to do more. I like my lessons simple and clear.

When I was 7 years old, my mother took my brother and I to visit a sick friend in the hospital. When we walked into the courtyard, there was an enormous concrete fountain with a large bird of some kind perched at the top. Water flowed out the bill and into the shallow pool below. Children were sloshing around in the water while their parents sat on nearby benches nestled under large maple trees. Glancing down at us, my mother said, "Behave yourselves when we go inside and I'll let you wade in the water for a bit before we leave."

When we emerged into the daylight, we were met with a hot Georgia breeze.

"Whew, I wouldn't mind taking a dip myself," my mother joked.

We shed our shoes and handed them to our mom. We cautiously straddled the warm concrete wall, testing the water to find it freezing cold, but anxiously went in. Wadding in the murky water we were careful to avoid some boys splashing and kicking about on the opposite side. I felt something under my feet; something round, smooth and slimy. My brother noticed it too, and together we reached down to feel. They moved about, they were all around our feet. I gasp, "Money!" I whispered to my sibling.

We scooped up all that we felt. "Do you think this is a wish pond?" I ask my brother.

"You betcha, sis. Look what I got," as he opened his hands to show me his find.

Holding the change in our hands, we wadded over to our mother who was sitting on the edge of the wall.

"Look mommy, we found a bunch of money. Someone rich must have tossed in this quarter!" My brother said as he held up the coin for inspection.

"Someone like us," my mother corrected. "Rich people only have nickel or penny wishes."

This was another one of her parables to teach me the value of life.

I left there empty handed, but wiser from the lesson. Most children don't pay attention to what their parents say, but I found my mother's words fascinating. She could explain certain things in my life in a way that I could understand. She spent exactly enough time on a subject to hold my interest. I listened and fit all the pieces together like a jigsaw puzzle. When despair seemed overwhelming, she could lose touch with the world or get up, brush off the dirt and raise her children and that's exactly what she did. I have no doubt that this woman from the hills of Kentucky with no college education could teach the world a few lessons.

5

The day finally arrives when I am recovered enough to go home. The excitement has my muscles twitching as I walk out into the bright daylight under a cloudless sky that seems to inflate the heavens. The air smells different, fresh and clean.

"It feels so good to be going home. I can't wait to see the kids."

"Yeah, and they can't wait to see you too," Philip replies.

I have devised a strategy to win this marathon. I have to keep my mind focused and not lose that drive to get my life back in order. Even though I have weathered most of the storm, I have to choose the right thoughts. I can't dwell over my problems, I am ready to continue my uphill climb. My life may not have turned out as I had hoped, but I know I can and will do this. With God's help I will.

As a child, I had a discouraging life. I allowed negative thoughts and words to infiltrate my mind, corrupting my forward movement. I could run, but I could not hide from all my pain and loneliness. My mother showered me with love and taught me how to live through diversity no matter what the situation. She gathered me under her wing, instinctively protecting me the best way she knew how. She taught me the power of prayer and to keep the faith through insurmountable circumstances. Now I need to make a conscious effort to follow her example. To realize the value of a mother, ask someone that has lost one.

"Mommy, mommy!" cries Haley as she runs out to greet me. The sight of her warms my heart. Something just clicked. I had faced a life-threatening situation and I survived. God is great, God is good. He is in the miracle working business, and by his grace I am alive and functional.

Haley climbs into my lap and wraps her arms around my neck for a big hug.

"Thank you Lord, this is what I need." I said out loud.

I hug my baby girl and cry uncontrollably. The sweetness of chocolate milk and fruity children's shampoo radiate from her. Her thin blonde wisp of curls tickle my nose. She looks like a little person instead of a toddler I left behind. Sara and Katie help me to my feet as I reach for my claw foot cane. In the arms of my children, I walk to the house.

"Please don't do this to us again," Sara whispers.

I'm proud of Sara for her willingness to care of her younger siblings. Although their grandparents were there, my children felt lost and out of their element. Sara knew her sister's unspoken needs and filled the void.

My life has become a constant struggle with the strain of rehabilitation, but I continue with relentless determination. I am not able to drive, so Bettye transports me to my appointments and physical therapy. I use a large wide elastic strap to exercise my left arm several times a day. Tied to the back of a chair, I pull the band from my shoulder to my lap. I do three sets of twenty reps. I want my life in control and don't like to be inconvenienced: I want things done right here and now, but I have to learn patience.

In the late evening, when the sun is on the horizon and the brunt of the heat is breaking, I enjoy sitting on the back patio and watch Haley drive her battery operated jeep around the perimeter of the yard while the older girls jump on the trampoline. This is the best time for free thinking. My mind drifts like clouds in an undecided breeze, taking first this direction and then the next. It's difficult for me to control my thoughts when I am tired. Thoughts of home, and more thoughts of my situation settle in. I don't want to sit back passively and expect God to do everything. After all it's the tough times in life that I find out what I'm really made of. I know God's using my husband, my family and even my children to be unwitting mirrors to reveal areas where I need to improve.

Looking back to my younger days, I remember when I was riding on the back of a motorcycle going to Grandfather Mountain in North Carolina. A car pulled out in front of us unexpectedly, so to avoid serious injury the driver laid the bike down. The driver let go and skidded to the side, but my leg was pined between the blinker and tail pipe. I was dragged under the two ton vehicle. The helmet ripped from my head, my leg forced upward parallel to my side with my foot under my chin. A wrecker raised the car off of me to allow the paramedics access. I thought that I would spend the rest of my life in a wheelchair. "Don't be afraid, the Lords with you. Fear is a lack of faith," my mother told me.

My trips to rehab gives me a change of scenery. It is good to be out of the hospital and home, but I still feel imprisoned. I missed my old life of multitasking with juggling work, kids and after school activities. I missed going to lunch with my friends and having the freedom to come and go at will. That's all changed now. It seems though, the more I go to physical therapy the less stressful it becomes. My progress is well received, and I push myself to get out of my comfort zone to avoid a pitfall. The stationary bike is my favorite. It works both my legs and arms at the same time. I'm able to compensate my weaker side better. Putt putt golf is my least manageable because I can't grasp the handle. It's hard to use my left hand to control the club.

Aside from physical therapy, I visit the Pearlman Cancer Center for my chemotherapy treatments and lab work. Dr. Anderson is extremely supportive and I feel comfortable airing my concerns with him. I suffer from a rare type of leukemia called Hypereosiniphilia. This is the cancer of the white blood cells instead of the red. These cancerous cells are mass produced in the bone marrow and spreads through the body infiltrating all organs. This build up eventually blocks needed blood supply which damages the organ. This clotting caused my strokes.

The chemotherapy treatments are for the most part tolerable. A small catheter is stitched into my right forearm for the sessions and any other type of intervenes medication the doctor orders. In addition to chemotherapy, Glevic (oral) and interferon (shot) is prescribed. Philip administers the shot in my thigh once a day. As the drug enters my body, it burns and is very painful. The shots leave tender welts that looks like a wasp sting. I know this is hard on him, but I can't bring myself to do it. As he rubs in injection site I see his sympathy in the form of tears.

He is so caring and would do anything for me, even take my pain if he could. He is a good listener, a person who can sit with me while I cry at a sad movie, or watch a chick flick and be compassionate about the worrisome burdens carried on my shoulders, the person who has the patience to watch a caterpillar crawl and to have patience with me. After awhile I learn to live with the pain, but I never get use to it.

I am given no approximate treatment time frame. I continue to take the drugs, shots, and chemotherapy regimen in the hope that my condition will improve and the hope of remission. I am under constant screening for any change.

Philip comforts me, "Don't worry about things. No big deal. Someday you'll realize that you don't have to fix everything that happens to you."

He is right. Many times I am tempted to fight a battle with my own strength like my mother did.

I want so badly to be able to pick up the phone and hear my mother's voice. To hear it from someone who has been there. I need to ask her how do I handle the times when life is like a torrential rainstorm, and each raindrop a test of my faith.

My mother is on my mind a lot. For years I could talk about her without crying. I would just sort of tick off the facts rationally like she was a distant relative, but when this all came about I get very emotional about her death. I have finally allowed myself to mourn my mother for the first time.

I remember in high school, I had to take one of those silly, insidious "what do you want to become" test. One question ask, if given a choice, would you prefer to do voluntary work at a hospital, visit a historical museum, or go to the lake. At 14, I didn't want to work in a hospital. It would be too depressing and a reminder of my own suffering. I had no money to spend on hours lingering around looking at priceless exhibits in a dimly lit museum. My honest answer was to go to the lake. When I got the test back, my answer was marked wrong. I remember the teacher saying something to the effect that I wouldn't amount to anything wasting my time with recreational things rather than getting some culture or helping the less fortunate. Even though he was trying to tell me to be more responsible, shape up, get serious, he didn't know that I was already beyond my years in experience.

My visits to Dr. Anderson reinforced my fight. He calms my fears with unbelievable sincerity.

"This is hard, disappointment will be a part of it, you've come back from the brink of death. You're in treatment for a rare disease and a cure won't happen automatically. It takes time. This is normal and expected." he explains.

I associate the cancer center with pain. Not only do I have chemotherapy treatments there, but bone marrow biopsies as well. This procedure is very painful.

I lay face down on an examine table and a local anesthesia is given in the small dimples of my lower back. The bone cannot be numbed. A hollow needle in inserted through an incision and on through the bone and into the bone marrow cavity. It is a deep aching pain when the needle is fully inserted. A syringe is used to draw a sample of the liquid portion of the bone marrow into the hollow needle. As the marrow is drawn up, I feel a stinging, pulling sensation which travels down my leg. The sample is checked to make sure it's adequate before the needle is removed. Then a different needle is inserted to collect a core sample of the bone. Afterwards a large pressure bandage is applied to help minimize the bleeding. This procedure is essential to provide Dr. Anderson detailed information on the condition of my blood cells and cancer count.

Since virtually everyone is aware of my situation, I use it as an opportunity for me to testify the power of faith and prayer. It's normally against my nature to talk so deeply and personally about things in my life. However, I know I am a miracle and feel the need to talk about my experience with anyone who will listen.

I am no stranger to prayer. I consumed most of my childhood praying for my father to change. My father would arrive home on many occasions intoxicated and someone or something would be the target of his anger. One vivid memory, I found it painful to ride a not so friendly Shetland pony that my father had won in a card game. Equipped with only a saddle blanket and a rope for a bridle, I climbed on it's back and braced myself for a rough ride. I squeezed my legs around the pony as he galloped to a crab apple tree at the far end of the field. Under the low branches of the tree, it bucked until his unwanted rider fell off. My father tethered and whipped the pony. Then with his feet dragging on the ground, he rode the pony until it submitted to weight on its back. I couldn't bear the sight of him abusing the animal, but in spite of it I was relieved that he had tamed it.

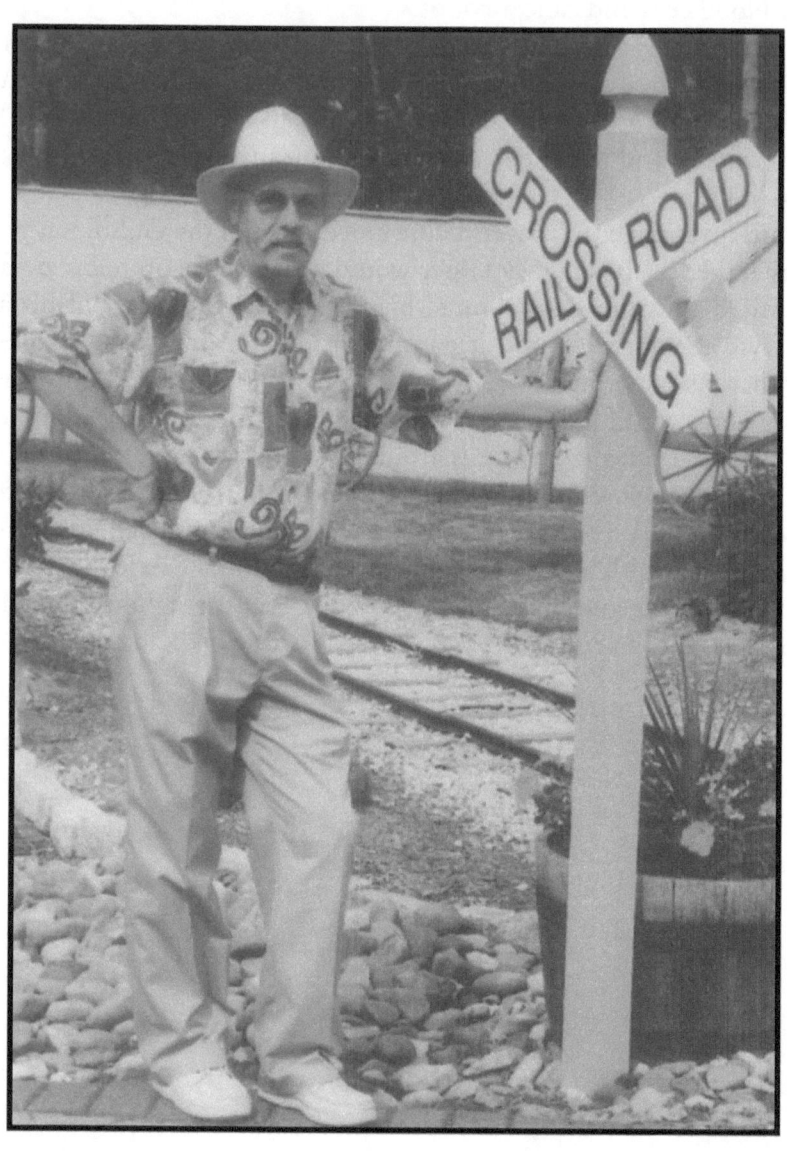

Daddy Don

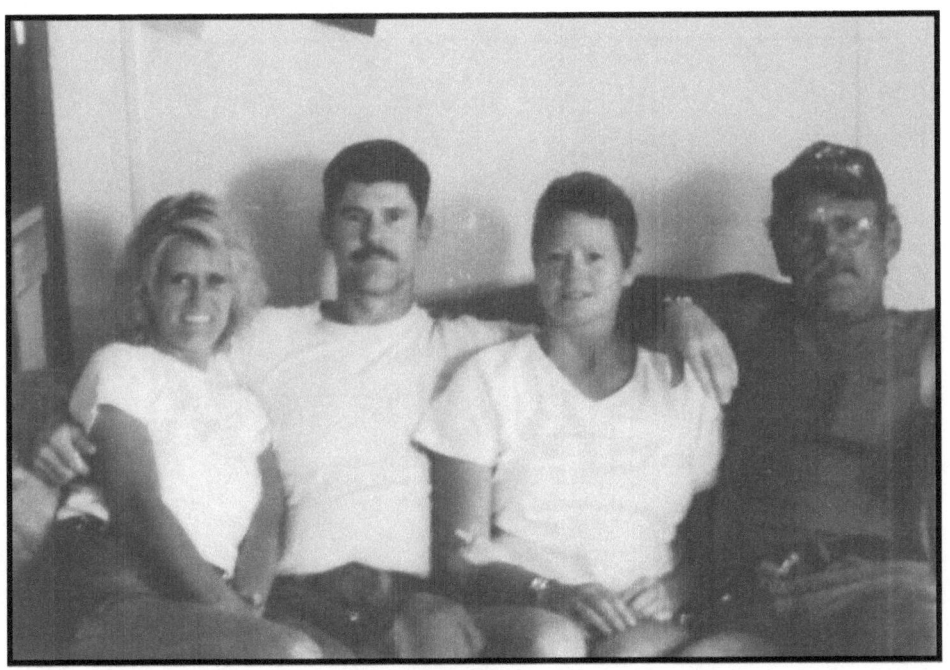

Diane, Dale, Me & David

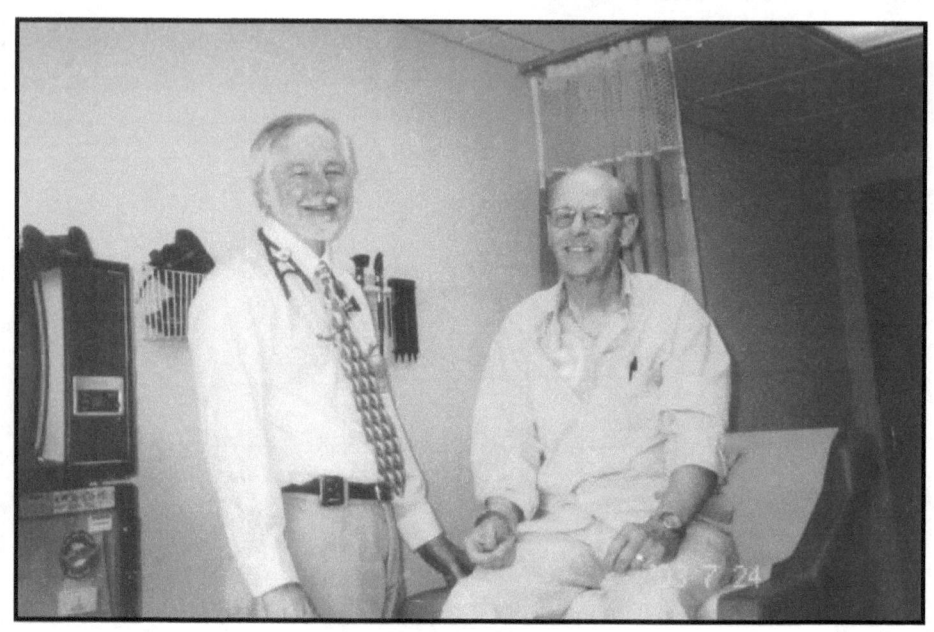

Dr. Wingard & Don

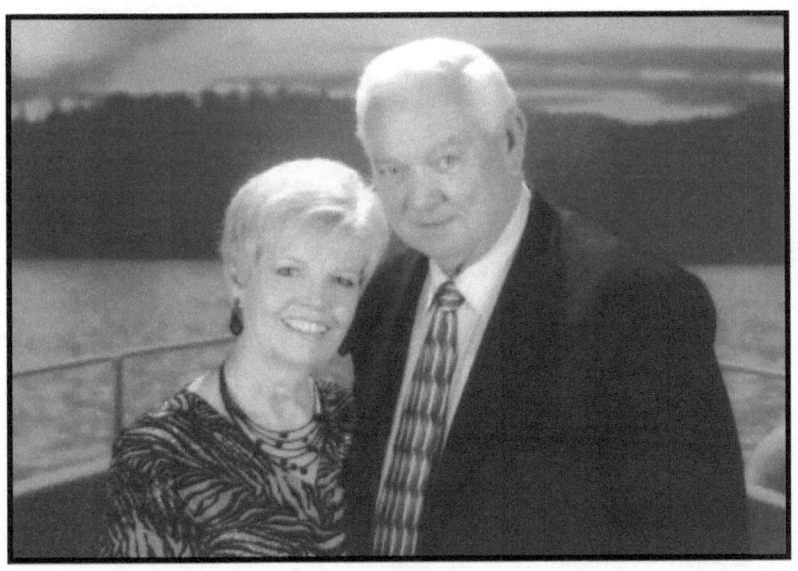

Mother & Father in-law, Bettye & Elton Keaton

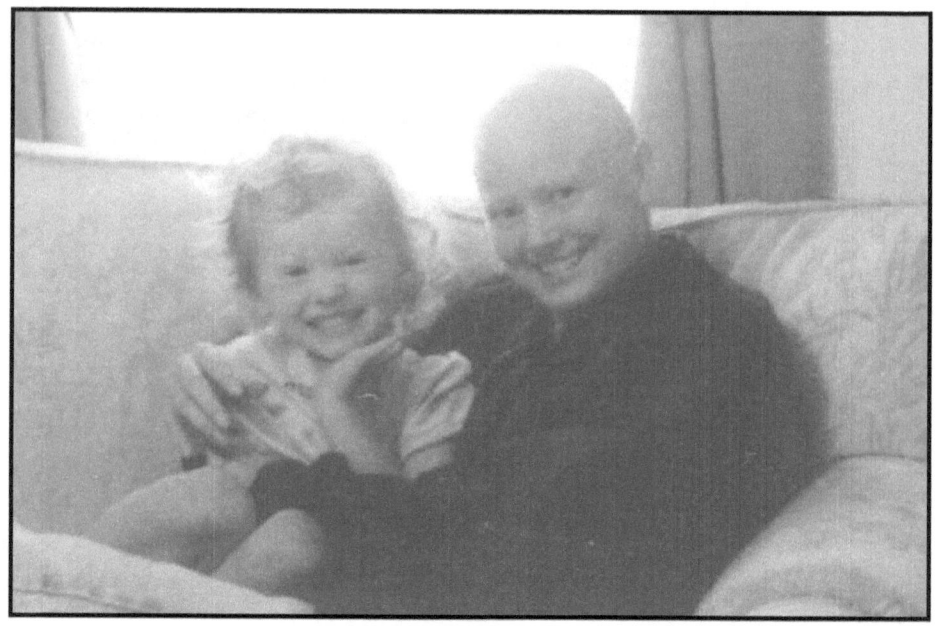

Haley with me in Transplant Housing

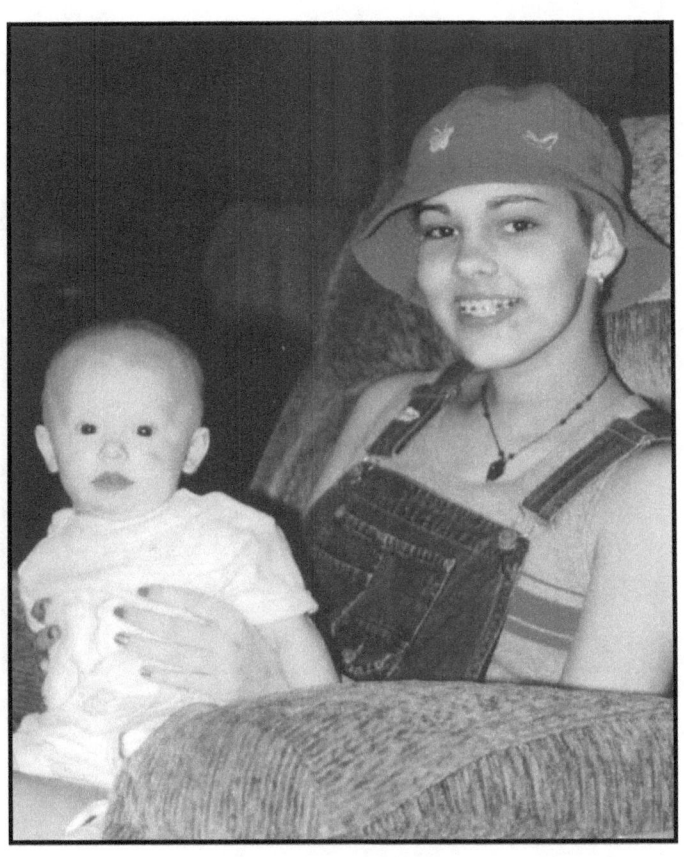

Jamie Day & Haley

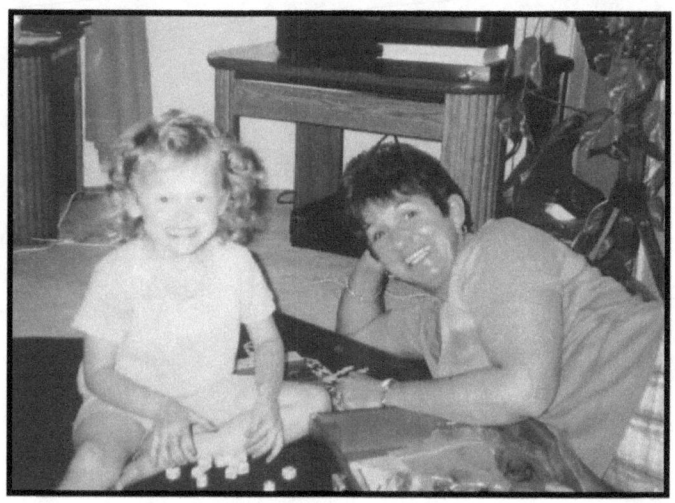

Boots visit to Transplant Housing

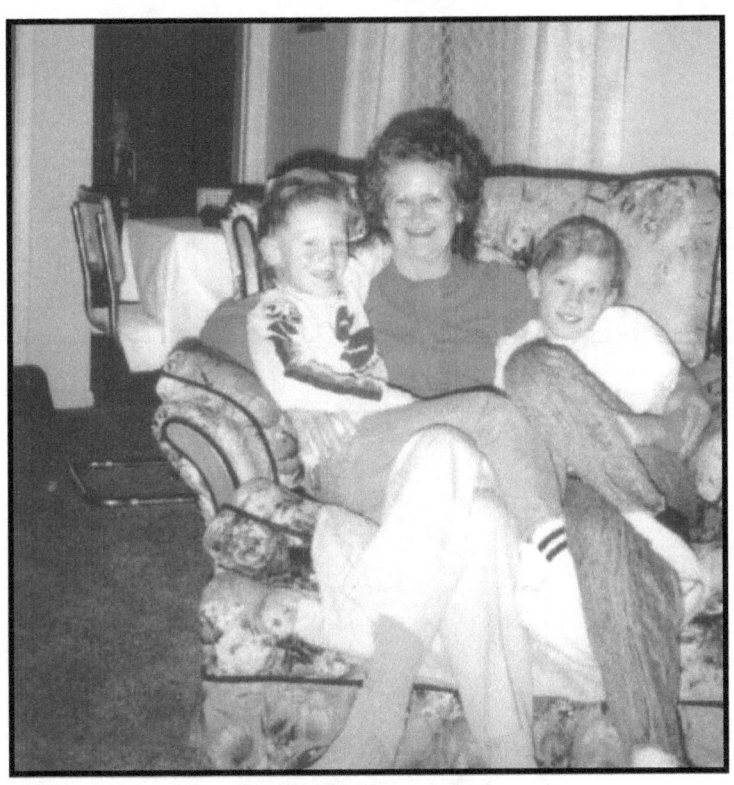

Josh, Katie (my mother) & Traci

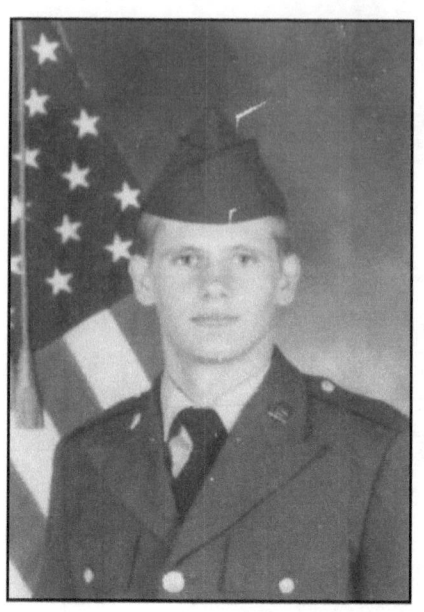

Ray

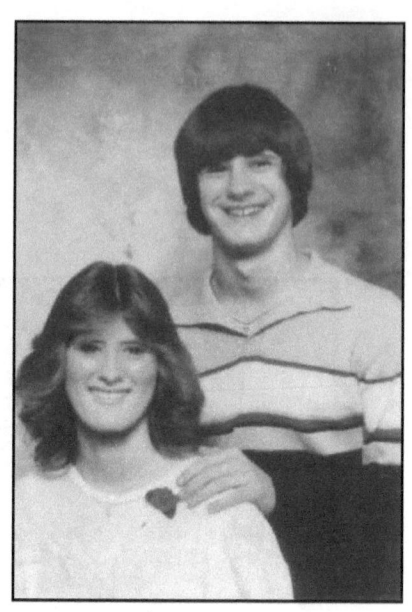

Mike & Marie

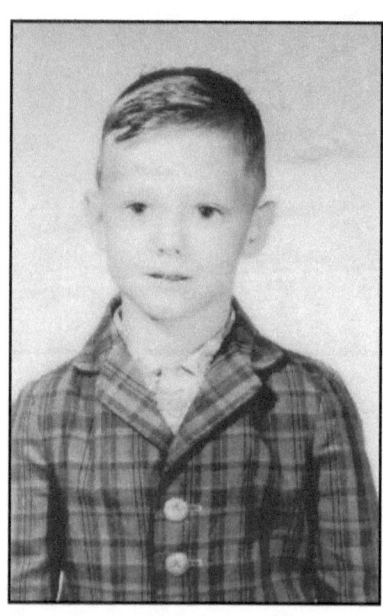

Chester

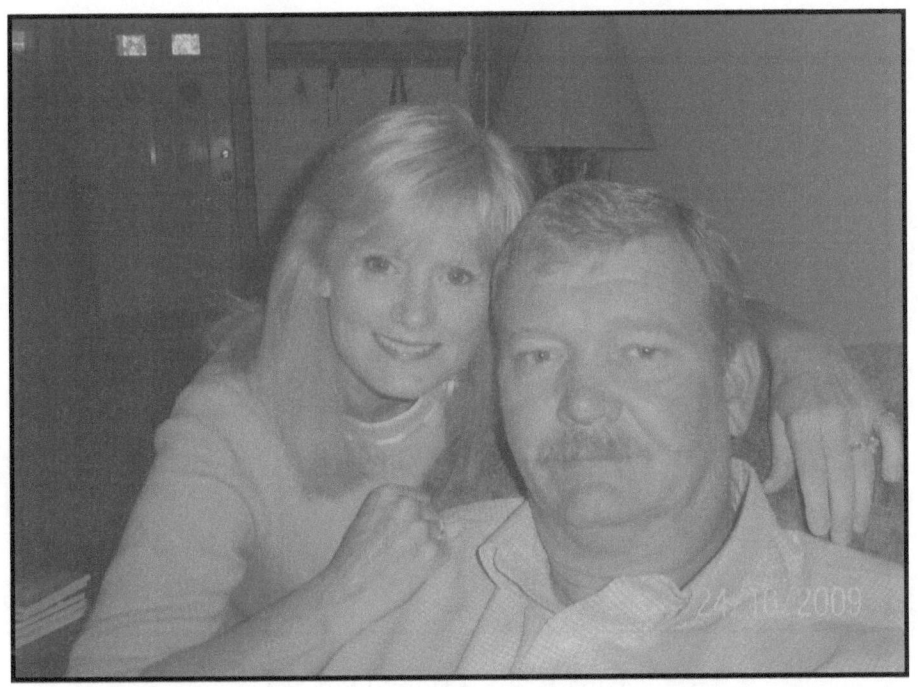

Lisa & Philip

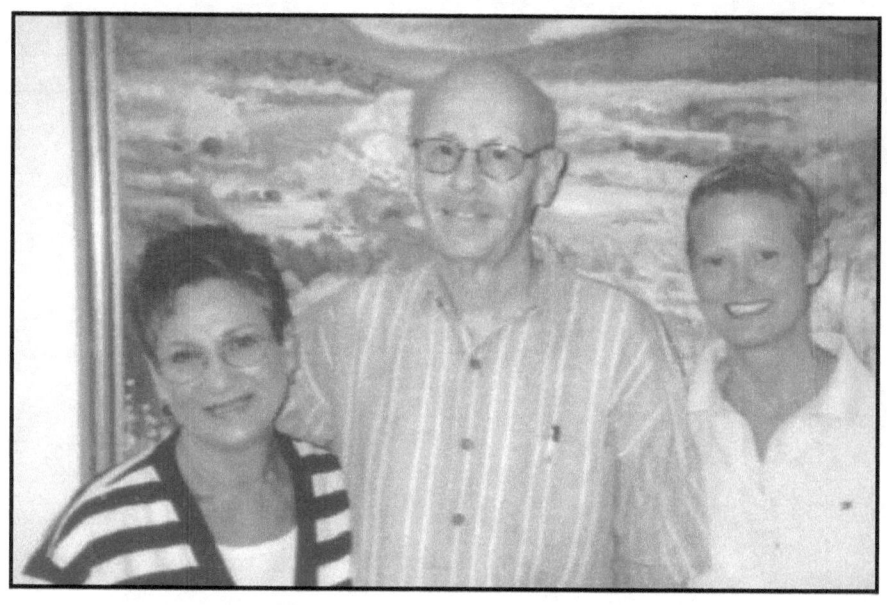

Mama Jackie, Daddy Don & I

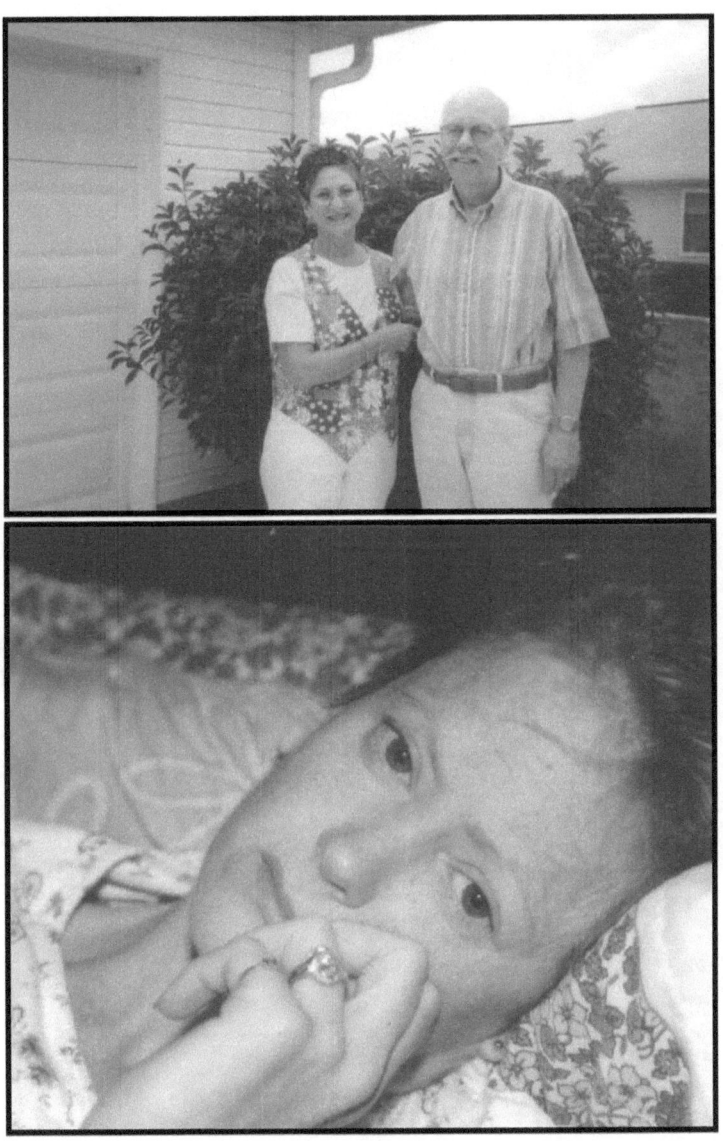

Me @ Shands and Don & Jackie Reuman (top)

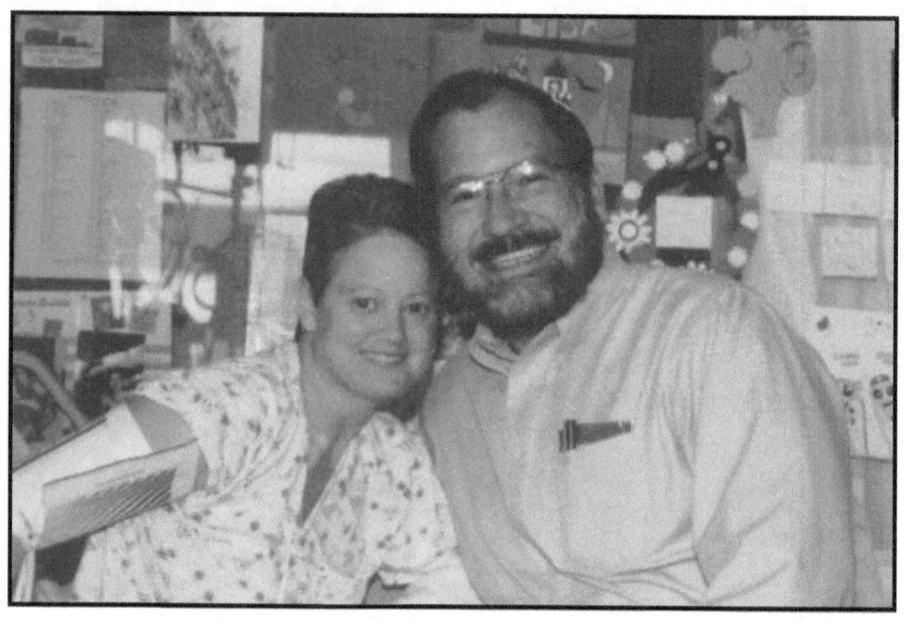

Me with Pastor Mickey Wisehart

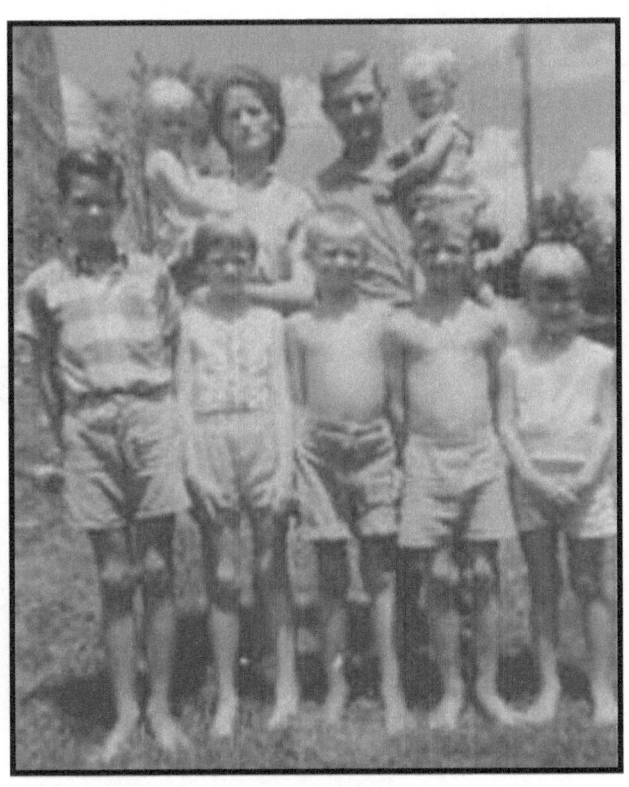

The Davidson's

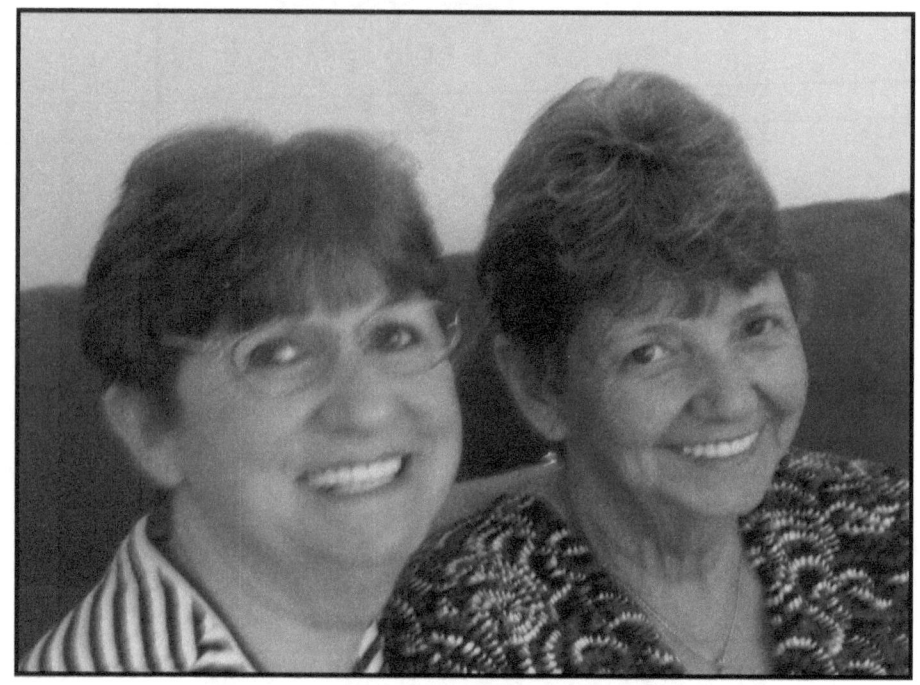

Boots & Jean

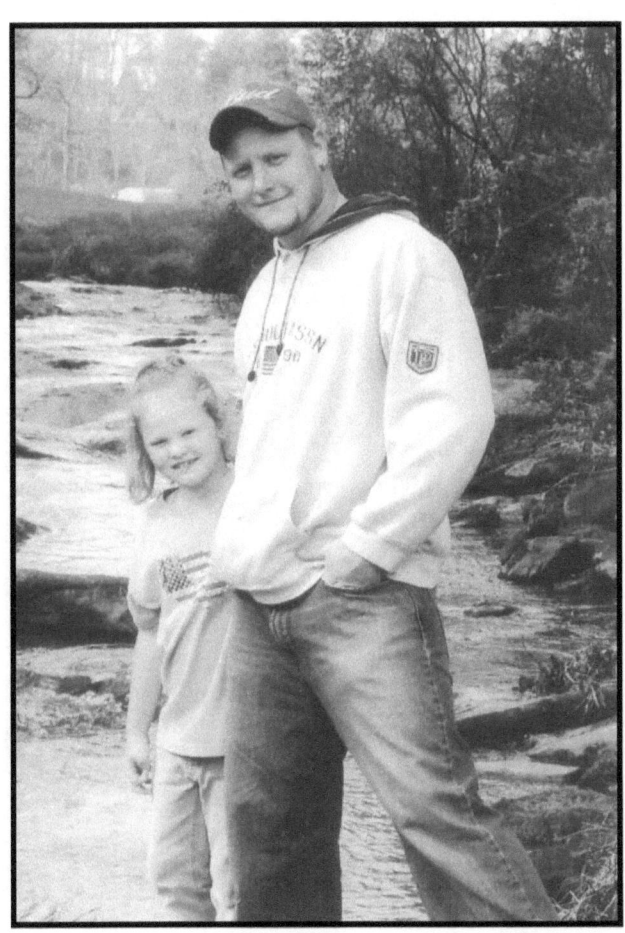

Haley & Joshua

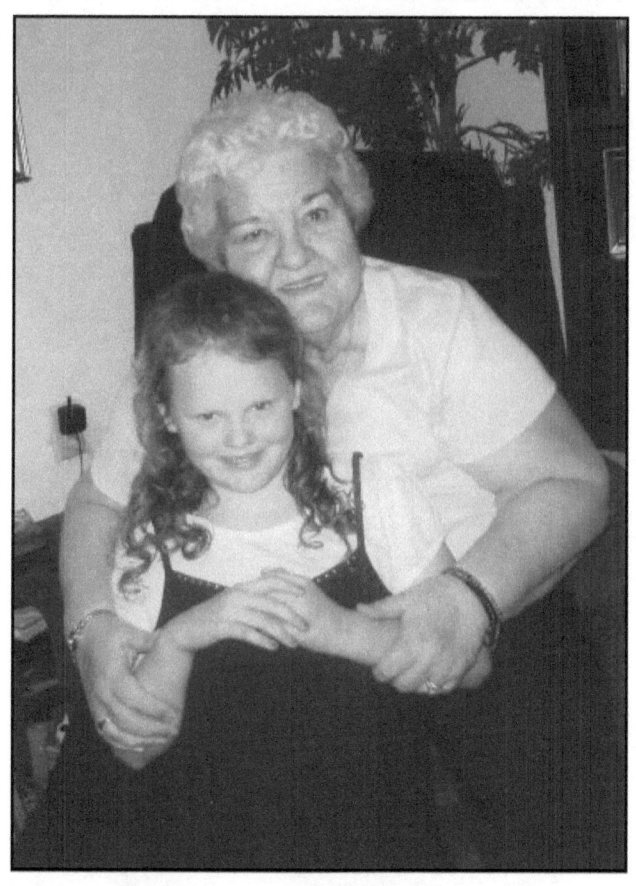

Haley & Nana Pat

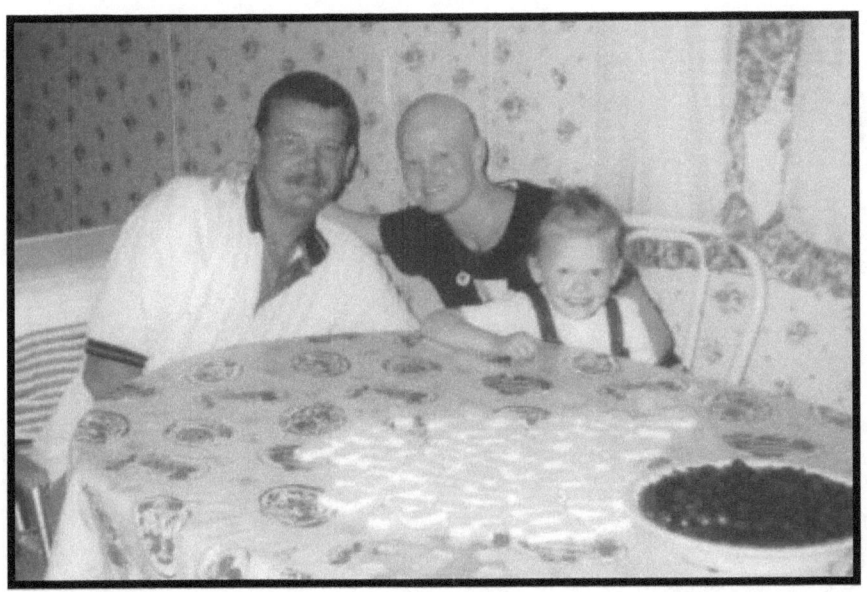

Playing Dominoes

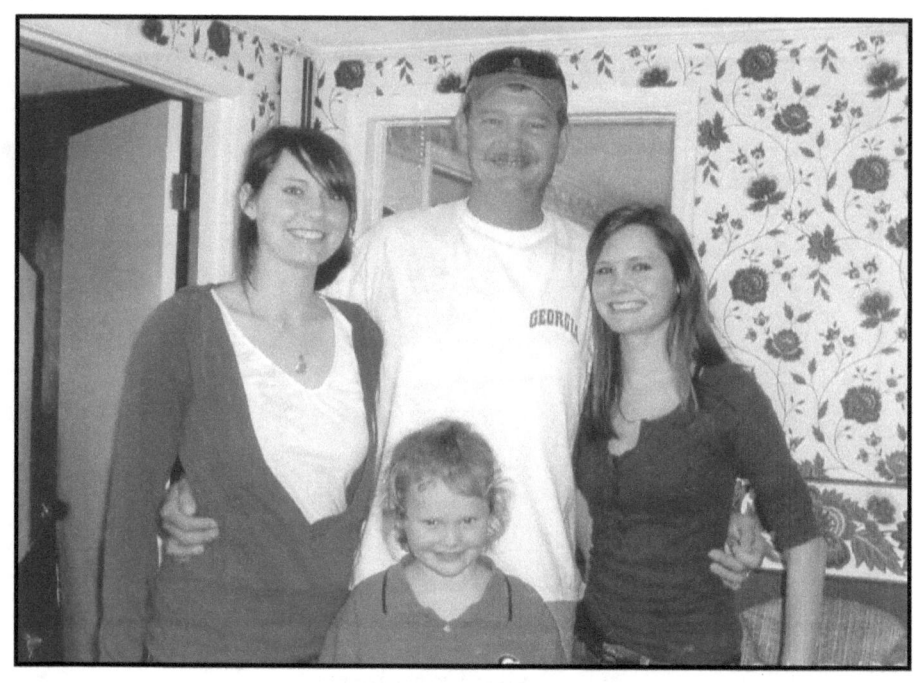

Sara, Philip, Katie & Haley

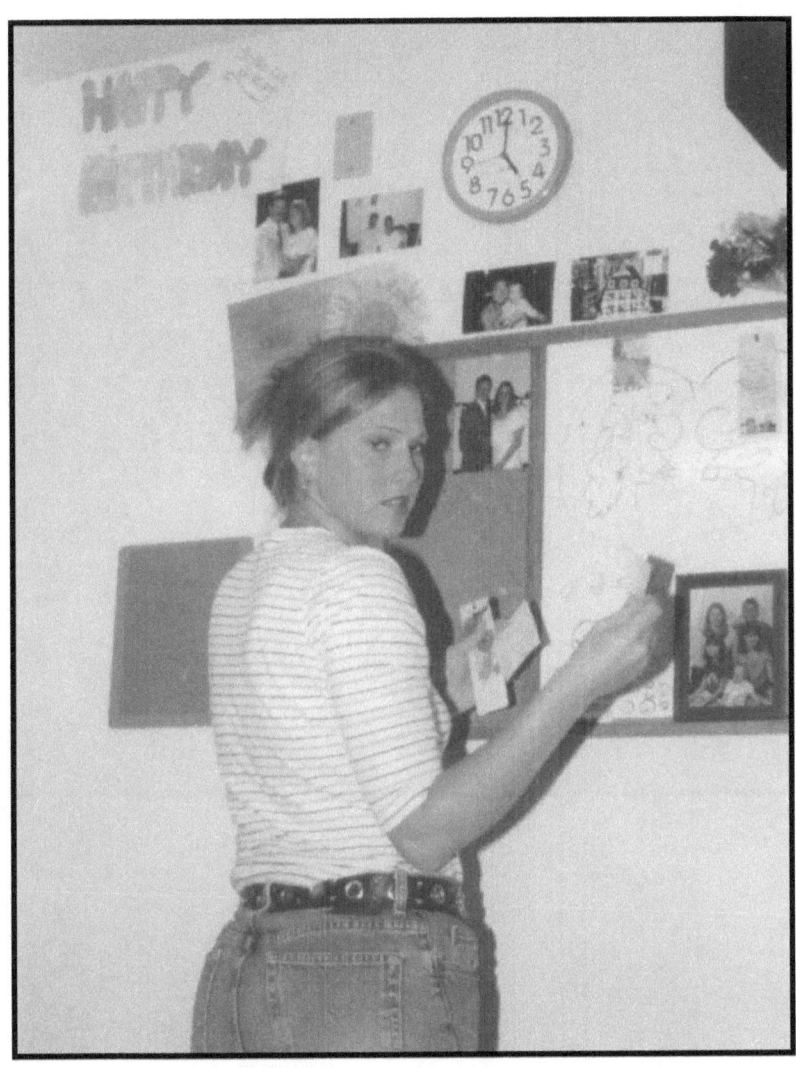

Traci visits me @ Shands

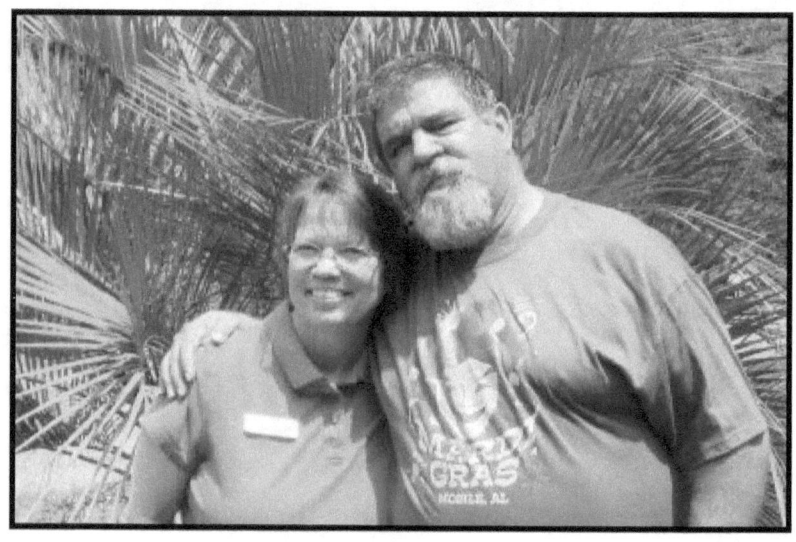

Sharon Butcher & husband Frank

6

A small, overly caffeinated nurse in a deep coral scrub, the color of ripe strawberries walks up to me sitting in a recliner receiving a chemotherapy treatment.

"Dr. Anderson would like to see you after we are done here. Okay?"

Philip and I walk across the hall to Dr. Anderson's office.

"Lisa, I've been on the phone with a specialist at Shands hospital and he has learned about a patient in Japan with the same blood disorder as you. A bone marrow transplant was tried with excellent results. The patient is showing signs of improvement and there is hope for remission from this cancer. Your progress with the chemotherapy, Glevic and Interferon is not what we expected. I'm aware that this is your decision, but I want you to let Shands help you. Your body can't keep going like this. Do you understand? This is your last chance."

Where do I start facing something like this. I keep telling myself to calm down and figure something out with logic and reason. After all, I'm not dead yet. Not yet.

"Doctor," I whisper, tightening my grip on the chair. "What is a bone marrow transplant? Is it bad? How bad?"

He didn't answer right away.

I drop my head and wring my hands in despair. "I guess this will be another human interest story."

"No," he interrupts.

I glance up.

"It's a story that needs to be written by someone who is a fighter, a survivor."

He leans back in his chair, its wooden joints heaving slightly. Then he drew himself straight, getting down to business.

"I'll make this quick." He takes a breath and begins.

I look at this man that is in his thirties. His hair is slightly long and shot with natural highlights, brushed back off his face as though with an impatient hand. I try to soak up what he is saying, but I really don't understand his words.

"I appreciate them, and I know they want to help, but a transplant? I'm scared."

"Scared? Listen to yourself. If you don't do this, you'll cheat yourself out of an opportunity of a cure."

His words shocked me. In my mind, I am trying to avoid any further punishment to my body. I am afraid that this will just be another failure.

"I'm just sick of being sick," I whisper.

Dr. Anderson hesitates a moment longer then reached for the clasps. The locks springs easily and he flips the lid open. The briefcase is full with a jumble of papers and none of them meaningful to me in any way. He moves his hand over it lightly, as if fearful of disturbing some unseen order. He removes several sheets of paper and hands them to me. It is as if someone had whispered my name from out of nowhere. For a moment I considered slamming his briefcase shut like I'd never been here, like I'd never seen this man.

Philip leans forward his elbows on his knees, studying my face, memorizing it for the suffering yet to come, and said.

"Yesterday you were told that you were dying, today you're still alive, tomorrow you will be healed. You need to try this, if not for yourself then for the kids and me."

With tears soaking up my face, "okay."

Lord, I don't know if I can go through anymore. I'm not sure I can do this.

A voice came to me, "Yes, you can."

The Lords words penetrate my consciousness. I feel renewed inner strength. I can't allow my mind to dwell on the biggest battle of my life. I need to focus on thoughts of life with joy and victory. The more I dwell on it, the more doubt Satan dumps into my mind, and will effect my emotions and my attitude. I know bad things happen to good people; I've lost my health, my job, and I am going through overwhelming financial burdens. I need to hold steadfast to my faith and stay emotionally healthy then the rest will follow. Jesus said, "In this life you will have trouble, but be of good cheer for I have overcome the world." I truly believe that he is greater than my problems. This is a tough test, the biggest test of my life, my faith and I don't want to fail.

I feel like David facing Goliath, looking small to a circumstance beyond my ability. The mountain of a man laughed when he saw a boy facing him, but David had someone much stronger than any weapon. He challenged Goliath in the name of the Lord. He didn't cower or hesitate. I need to stop worrying about how big this cancer is and challenge it with my faith. My positive attitude will renovate my soul, my outlook, my belief that even today God is still in control.

After we leave the cancer center, Philip and I drop in to see my co-workers at the University post office.

"My oncologist says that there's a possible cure for me."

"Really?" ask Amanda.

There are smiles and cheers from everyone in the office.

"God bless you!" Ted says.

Ted Davis and Amanda Williams have been employed at the campus post office for almost as long as myself. They have the tedious task of delivering the mail and packages to all the campus offices and return with outgoing mail to be metered. As Assistant Manager, I worked alongside the staff and yet earn their respect. This includes my six part time student assistants as well. I enjoyed my job, and I felt comfortable helping customers or handling the mail. Even though Sharon is the backbone of the office, It is my responsibility to reinforced the policies and procedures, thus keeping a harmonious environment.

During the morning ritual of casing mail, if someone was having a bad day, I would make a light hearted comment like "I'm happy to be here. Everyday is a bonus day!" Everyone would respond with a hearty "Amen!"

"I sure needed to hear that," said the grumpy employee.

The University staff are like family, and the news of the transplant spreads like wild fire throughout the system. Sharon creates a web site with pictures and information about the search for a donor. The web site list the organizations to contact for possible donor screening. She organized a fund-raisers, sold T-shirts printed with the logo "Fundraiser For Lisa". A lady donated a handmade quilt to auction off. The quilt was absolutely beautiful and thankful that a stranger would offer something so time consuming to help me. Everything sold through all events, T-shirts sales and donations were deposited into a separate account for my transplant. The web site also generated support and was updated regularly to insure constant funding. Sharon was pure in heart with everything she did for me. Some hopes fail to deliver. Some expectations sputter and flop like an untied balloon and you know when you're at the end of the rope, but this all was surreal with so much compassion and giving in my community. I felt so loved.

I continue taking a garden variety of medications to help control the cancer count and endure the painful interferon injections, but I worry that my time would run out before a suitable donor was found. I don't want to die. Not yet. I want to see my kids fulfill their dreams. *Please, Mama, if you've still got that pipeline to the man upstairs, ask him to give me a break. I know you told me that "worry is a lack of faith," but I'm human with flaws way to many to count. I keep reminding myself that God will give me what I need, not what I want.* Even though this is confusing, I have to keep in mind that God sees the big picture. I have to trust him and try not to fear what I can't see. He's getting all the ducks in a row and in *his* time it will all come together.

We are shocked when the cancer center social worker finds out that my insurance policy rendered useless. My health plan excluded risky, experimental treatments. In other words, it did not cover the DNA/HLA testing which is a critical and expensive aspect of care. I could not have a transplant without a donor, I am forced to pay out-of-pocket for the search. Philip gives the bone marrow transplant coordinator a credit card and said,

"When it maxes out, let me know."

At a cost of $850 per candidate for HLA high-resolution tissue typing, the card quickly reaches the credit limit. Another card is handed over and it too is maxed out. In total, three credit cards are to the limit and a second mortgage is taken out.

The onset of the donor search, it was discovered that a sibling matched six of ten antigens but unfortunately she had hepatitis C. The transplant team felt that in my weakened state I might not be able to fight off the infection, so the decision is made to continue the search and only use the sibling if no other option is available. The transplant searches through thousands of registries all around the world, but after an exhausting four month screening, only a few passed the initial stage, but failed the final DNA test. In the end another twenty donors are typed free of charge because the transplant coordinator enrolled me in a study sponsored by the National Marrow Donor Program, which also failed. With time an essence, the head of the transplant program and professor of the Department of Medicine and the Division of Hematology and Oncology, Professor John R. Wingard, has no choice but to use my sibling, despite the risks.

It is of great significance to have this transplant as soon as possible while I am still physically able to withstand the process. I spend a week at Shands for labs, conferences and screening. I am amazed how meticulous the transplant team is in the state-of-the-art test, leaving no stone unturned.

I have never been subjected to so much attention. It is like I am the only person to ever go through this. I seem calm on the surface, but underneath I am deeply affected. My stomach knots at the thought of how I desperately want to live. *Buckle in, it's going to be a another rough race, but when I cross that finish line, I will get a gold medal.*

Sensing my anxiousness, Philip says to me, "Believe in yourself, Lisa. Believe in the power of the Lord. Let him do his job."

"I'm sorry, I can't help but be scared."

"We've got to trust him. He's saved you once already and he has the power to do it again." he whispers.

"Okay."

Over the next several weeks, I get all loose ends taken care of. I have a will drawn up and contact my distant family. Philip works long hours to enhance our savings so it will help while he is with me during the toughest time.

On the 16th of February, I gather my children around and tell them it is time for me to leave. I ask Sara to help her grandmother take care of her sisters. Traci who lives nearby reassures me that she will also be there for her siblings. I hug my children as we pray for me to return to the person I was before cancer conquered my body. In my mind, I can see myself running and playing with my kids again. *Lord help me have hope no matter the circumstances.*

I keep my composure until we are out of sight and then I loose it. I feel guilty for leaving and disrupting the routine again.

My mind is filled with visions of my mother suffering in the final days of her life and Philip's young cousin Jamie dying at the age of sixteen. I am tempted to hold on to the hurt and pain of seeing who I loved dearly leave this earth. God, help me quit mourning over what has been lost; I know doing this will restore my life. *If I die will Haley remember me?* I don't want her to miss out on knowing her mother. I want to be able to share my life stories slowly, meting them out as they deem appropriate for her current developmental stage. I don't want to die and take my stories with me, leaving her to reconstruct them whatever way she can. When she gets older and looks in the mirror and see my face, hands and feet; it will be like her body unfolding to a paper-doll image of me.

Lord, don't shut those elevator doors just yet. My kids need to give their mother another hug.

7

As our Jeep Cherokee travels down the all to familiar stretch of Interstate 75, Philip slides my favorite CD Traci burned for me in the player. I close my eyes and stretch out my legs for the two hour drive. I feel somewhere different. I am quiet and introspective when I have always been self-sufficient and well grounded before.

In my high school days, I threw myself into my studies, classes were lively, I was taking all the typical high school courses such as History, English, Biology, and Spanish. I had no time or money for extra curricular activities. I worked help my brother Dale support the family.

After graduation, he enlisted into the Marine Corps and he gave me his cherished Chevy Camaro for transportation. I accepted the gift with a secret promise to return it when I no longer needed it. Though at times it was a lot to deal with I accepted the fact that this was the way it was, but sometimes it was just too overwhelming, and crying released tremendous tension. God created tear ducts as a pressure release valves and mine operated just fine. I found comfort in my mothers words on those occasions. She would tell me a story to ease my frustration and lift me up, and they always blended in with that particular situation.

This was a story she told me about two brothers walking up to some out of town kids and asking to play.

"Sure," said the big kid standing with his arms crossed, "if ya'll race me up that hill."

The older brother points to the big kid, himself, to his sibling and then to the hill covered with loose gravel and dirt. The younger weaker brother nods and the race was on. As the boys scrambled up the hill a boy on the ground yelled, "its to hard, ya'll will never make it." Among laughter, another boy shouted, "no chance that scrawny one will last. It's to high!" About half-way up, fighting the loose dirt, the older brother collapsed. The kids continued to yell, "Wahoo! One down! No one will make it; just give up." A short distance more, the big kid slid down. To tired, he also quit. But the puny one kept on going higher and higher. It was like he had a second wind and he wouldn't stop until he reached the top. One of the kids ask how he found the strength? His brother smiled and said, "he's deaf and couldn't hear you putting him down." Through her comforting stories, she was able to help me deal with the pressures I faced.

"God will help you through this. He will help us all." My mama said.

She had never held a job outside the home because of so many children. I never blamed her for our misfortune. I watched her swallow her pride and accept food and clothing donations from soup kitchens, charities, welfare, and food stamps to provide for her family.

For the most part we were healthy children. The only physical concern I encountered was at sixteen years old, my mother took me to the emergency room for a severe bout of vomiting. We had no health insurance, so I was treated for a stomach virus and sent home. After four hours of uncontrolled vomiting we returned to the hospital and this time admitted for an emergency appendectomy. I was back to school and my job in a few days.

"You're not here are you?" Philip ask.

"What do you mean?"

"You're lost in thought. You're somewhere else, I think." He glanced at me. "Somewhere better."

I nod and look towards the heavens. "Today is stressful for me. I ought to be home with my children. Haley's only a toddler and needs her mother.

When I was young, I would chase after my brothers across fields of tall grass. Smelling pine trees and listening to the sound of a wide, winding stream on its journey to Lake Lanier. I thought that owned the world. I would sit in a half-hearted fort made of limbs and pine straw, and imagine that we were Indians around a fire writing in the sand, the plans of the next buffalo hunt. My brother Ray would pinch off the end of fire flies to smear on his face for war paint. We would play for hours in the crisp night air until my mother called us in. I always had my mother close to me. As I got older and times were more difficult, I searched for my own identity, my self worth. The most I remember about my father is the smell of butane lighter fluid and alcohol, but I worked alongside my mother at eight years old as she taught me how to cook, can vegetables, and do the laundry. I cut my brothers hair and trimmed my sisters. You could say I had more responsibilities than the average child my age. Then years later, I saw you standing against the sloping side of a truck, your arms crossed, tall, lean, dirty blonde hair, and transparently, soulfully happy. I wanted to be like that. After what seemed a lifetime of disappointments I finally found what I was looking for. You rescued me and made my life complete.

"Remember our first date?", I ask Philip.

"Yep, I do. I took you to Tallahassee to watch the submarine races. I parked alongside a large pond with a fountain in the middle. I spread a blanket out near the water. For several minutes we sat in silence looking out over the water. So, do you like the races? I ask you. We laughed so hard. I like hearing you laugh. Seeing you happy, makes me happy."

We arrive at Shands in the late afternoon. The February wind is brisk blowing in from the northwest, promising a chilly night. I draw a large breath of fresh air as if is my last.

"We're here," I said dreadfully.

"I love you. You'll do just fine. I'll be with you every step of the way."

He takes my hand. I hold his tight. "I love you too."

Despite all the conferences and reading I had done, I still feel ill-prepared for this. I wished to be anywhere but here. I watched my mother suffer for years with breast cancer before she succumbed to the decease. I did not want my family to witness that with me. I did not want Philip to helplessly watch me waste away. I love Him so deeply. We never had to struggle with the idea of "love". It had come early, and easily, and often. We said it giddily to each other as if in high school it was said over the phone, and email. I would find notes in my lunch bag, "I love you" in my purse.

Standing silent in the elevator I strain to figure out what had gone wrong-what else could I have done to prevent this.

Looking up at Philip, "I'm not ready. We've not really talked about this, but there's one thing I need from you."

"Umm, what" he ask softly.

"No matter what happens, I want you to promise me that you'll grow old with someone special."

He turns me around and incased my face in his hands.

"Listen to me. I'm growing old with the person God's given me and I'm looking at her. How does that sound?"

Instantly I imagined him a rumpled old man in a ragged navy jean jacket with wildly sprouting white hair and a mustache. His hands shaking slightly, lost in thought, working on his fishing rod and reel. I want so desperately to stay a part of his world.

Sitting across from an impressive mahogany desk with a jumble of documents yet to be filed, I watch this slightly overweight woman with bad skin highlight sections and checks places to sign.

"You're all set," she says and gathers the papers up; taps them down to align them. "You can go on up to the fourth floor where someone will be waiting for you."

I walk up to the door of room 424 and stand outside reluctant to go any further. Philip takes my hand and ushers me inside. At first, I find it a place of dead energy. It is large, cool and fragrant. Inside the main entry is another much larger one covered with wide plastic strips hanging from the ceiling with hard burst of air blowing down like in the entrance of some department stores. The rest of the wall is plexiglass. Behind the bed the wall is covered with air filter panels that emits a humming sound as it continually empties the room of germs and dust.

"I'm not going to be able to sleep with all this noise," I moan under my breath.

Hanging in the corner overlooking the five foot window is a nice size television with working speakers. The small cream colored tile bathroom completes my world for the next six to eight weeks. I will be isolated from the outside world, no visitors, only phone calls, mail and my laptop until post transplant.

I cautiously sit down on the bed to test its firmness as Philip looks out the window. Down below are muted bleats of car horns and the occasional burst of shouting, as if an entire rolling ocean away.

"This is it," I said.

"This is it," he repeats, though neither of us really knew what "it" meant.

Soon an orderly arrives to take me for my catheter placement. I sit stiff in the wheelchair as I am wheeled to the surgical ward. Like a security blanket a sheet covers my legs and blue hospital socks. I receive warm glances from women in pink uniforms, red vest and striped pinafores cradling mail and care packages to patients.

The room is cold and noisy. The technician seems oddly nervous as I am. I feel like a lamb to the slaughter and can't do anything about it. He looks young, but beyond his years in experience not just an employee who happened to be in this room with me. To my left I see photographs, X rays, and slides of my chest. He injects something into my IV and suddenly, I am warm, numb, and very relaxed. Within a few minutes the surgeon walks into the room with a serious aura about him. He's a medium built man with straight brown hair, black slacks, and long-sleeved white shirt under his lab coat.

"This won't take long, it will be over soon," said the doctor.

Although groggy, I feel pressure as an incision is made just below the collar bone and the catheter is passed under the skin yet above the muscles. It is then stitched into an artery that leads to my heart. I feel a tugging sensation as he completes the procedure. In forty-five minutes, I am brought back to the transplant ward on a gurney.

"Hi there. You going to sleep all day?" a familiar voice says.

"Yeah, I'm going to sleep through this whole thing."

Something feels extremely tight over my collar bone. I glance down at the pressure bandage. Blood seeping slowly into the gauze. I feel a dull ache, like I'd been hit by something. The rest of the day, I lay in bed watching TV. I know that it is the calm before the storm.

February 19, 2003 starts with a delicious breakfast. "Not bad for hospital food, huh?" I said between bites.

"Yeah, it's pretty good." Philip replies.

Since the caregivers are constant fixtures until the patient leaves the transplant ward, they get a meal served also.

Chemotherapy begins two hours later. If I only knew that breakfast would have to last for ten days, I would have savored every bite. The treatments are every four hours around the clock for a week. It takes two hours to administer a unit and then a two hour break before it starts over again. This continues until the day before the transplant. I'll get one day to rest, if that's the right word.

On the beginning of the second day, I wake with my pillow covered with hair. The back of my head is completely bald. A nurse offers clippers if I want Philip to buzz what's left on my head, but I can't bring myself to let him do it. I know trying to keep my hair is a lose-lose situation. I know it will only be a short time before it is all gone anyway.

My appetite already suffering, Philip asks,

"You have to try to eat something, how about I get you a plain baked potato. Will you eat then?"

He heads for the door, only to have it pushed open before he reaches for the handle. Stepping back, he groans inside. His blue eyes narrowed slightly.

"Again already?"

With a stiff grin, she shakes her head. "This is just for starters. I'm sorry."

I grit my teeth and through tight lips, "This is the worst you have to dish out?"

The third day, my head is slick as a baby's behind. My head circumference measures only nineteen inches; I look like a bald child. I grow increasingly uncomfortable with the buildup of chemicals in my body. It gets harder to keep the feeling of sickness with an inclination to vomit at bay. A push of the call button summons anti-nausea shots which are generously given.

By the forth day, blisters form in my mouth and down my throat to my stomach. I can not swallow anything. I am fed fluids, blood transfusions, and medication for nausea through the IV. One night a transfusion of two units of blood is ordered. The first unit is administered with no complications, but I have a reaction to the second. At one in the morning, halfway through the bag, I wake with my throat closing up. I manage to squeak out a call for help. In an instant, help is summoned and a team of first responders are in the room. A large male nurse effortlessly moves the plexiglass wall to allow easy access. As I claw at my throat, the nursing staff urgently encircle my bed, each doing something different.

"Hold on." A nurse assures me. "We're going to get you out of this. I know it's a scary, but try to relax and let us help you." I am terrified, but oddly feel safe at the same time. She disconnects the IV while another nurse gives me several shots to halt anaphylaxis shock. I feel like my lungs are exploding from the pressure. I am horrified at the feeling of suffocation. The nurse claps an oxygen mask to my face and I gulp in air, lightheaded with relief. There's constant communication, talking me through my ordeal. Three minutes pass one click at a time. I sit upright in bed, panting for a breath. The rest of the night, Philip watches me, his elbows on his knees, resting his chin in his hands not knowing how to ease my suffering. He feels confident now that they could handle themselves in an emergency, no matter the situation.

Philip is there to wipe my face and neck with damp cloths. He's there to help the nurse change my vomit soaked gowns. He's there to console and support me. He takes care of me like an overly protective parent and not once does he complain.

He brings my hand up to his mouth and kisses it.

"Thank you for putting up with me." I whisper.

"There's nothing to put up with," he says.

"I know I get lost in myself sometimes."

"So do I, sweetie. You're like a kite blowing in the wind and God's holding the string to keep you from plummeting to the ground. You are a mess right now, miserable and so sick, but it's got go happen for you to get better. Don't be afraid."

"I'm just sick of being sick." I mumble.

The thought of suffering like my mother had, dug a hole down inside me and filled it brimful with fear-a ripping, tearing fear that infected my joy when I allowed myself to think about it. My brothers David, Dale and I stood at my mother's bedside as she took her last breath. I never got over the look of her once vibrate blue eyes now a dim gray in a face so thin and tiny that it seemed you could see right through her. I caressed her hand that was so cold and nails blueish purple. The hospice nurse told us that the hearing is last to go, so we each leaned over and kissed her goodbye and told her how much we loved her and it was okay for her to go be with her three boys. It has been years since she passed away, but I still miss her terribly.

As the days crawl by, it seems at times too much to bear. Some minutes better than others. I look as white as the sheet on which I lay. All I want to do is nothing, absolutely nothing. My misery has consumed my being.

"You okay?" Philip wipes my mouth.

"No. I sound less than gracious, but how long can one vomit like this? It has been so long without getting sick. Will it ever end?" I shake my head carefully, since that seems to aggravate the pressure headache that hover at the edges of my eyes. Extra anti-nausea medication is administered that brings some relief. I don't count days; I don't count hours; I count minutes.

February 26, finally arrives and I receive my sisters stem cells harvested earlier that morning. Since I was admitted some fifteen days ago, I have dropped from one hundred twenty five to a mere ninety six pounds. My last chance for a new life is brought in a regular not so special looking IV bag. It is a beautiful orange color with pink pearl swirls. *How could something so small give so much. It's more precious than all the riches in the world!*

"Happy birthday mama, this is your second birthday," Traci says through a mask.

"Thank you baby, but it's my third. My second is when I was baptized. I've been born again twice now."

"And you have the Lord to thank for all three." Philip says, as he and Traci watch this gift of life flow in to my body. Traci and I make a birthday poster with the date and tape it on the wall. The one hundred day post transplant countdown begins the next day. The calendar under the television marks off the days completed. I am so weak from the trauma to prepare for this, I want nothing but sleep. *It would have been a whole lot easier for me if they had put me to sleep until today. I couldn't eat, and only suffered anyway, so what's the difference?*

That night I lay in bed and look at the star canopy arched above me. The full silver moon hung in the sky with a twinkling star dangling off the lower point, as if caught like a fish. Smiling to myself, I begin to reminisce to Philip about a trip to visit my family in Kentucky when I was a child.

"I found my uncle Hargus in the barn on his knees rubbing his milk cows belly. I ask him what he was doing and he said, "Bell's been laboring too long. She needs help with the calf." I could see the calf's front hoofs showing. My uncle crawled around and grabbed the calf's legs and pulled. I watched as the calf slid out onto the ground, still encased in the birth sac. My uncle picked up some nearby straw and scrubbed the sac away, clearing the muzzle. It shook its head at the intrusion and bleated, coughing up phlegm. While it lay still for a moment, helpless, gaining strength, Bell surged to her feet, then turned and licked her baby.

"Whatcha gonna to with that calf?" I ask.

"Well, if he turns out big. I'll breed 'em. If not then I'll send him to slaughter." he replied.

I was so relieved to see that calf grow into a massive bull. You know, I feel helpless like. "

I will have to stay in the bone marrow unit for two weeks more before I move into transplant housing. I always wear a mask when I venture outside my room. Even though it's still on the ward, I fear that I'm accessible to infection. Philip encourages me to get out and explore the many halls of the transplant ward. He shows me the large snack room with vending machines, and an exercise room with stationary bikes covering two walls and treadmills in the center.

"I can't imagine anyone on this floor able to use this stuff, especially me." I joke.

Down one hall is a huge sitting area with large spacious windows with an impressive display of potted plants decorating overstuffed sofas and recliners.

"I come in here sometimes when you're sleeping to read or watch T.V. Now that you can get out of your room a little bit, we'll walk down here to have a change of scenery." He says.

"I've grown to like my room and feel safe where no dirt or germs dare to reside, but I promise I will start walking the halls with you. Right now, I just want to lie down. My knees are shaking, I'm still so weak,"

My life has presented a new set of challenges. Was it something in particular I could have done to prevent this? I think everyone asks this question with an accident or major illness, and in the end we are as lost for an explanation as before.

8

Now in transplant housing, I feel leery about being away from my germ free environment at the hospital. My bedroom is more like a motel room, but it's a step up from the noisy place I called home for so long. I am in a delicate post transplant stage. I lack physical strength or energy, and vulnerable to infections. Transplant housing permits close monitoring for signs of rejection or infections that may arise. Three times a week, my day begins with lab work at the BMT (Bone Marrow Transplant) ward. Eight to ten tubes of blood are drawn from the port in my chest to check my blood count and determine treatment. Extra tubes are used for the research program I enrolled at the beginning of this ordeal.

Once diagnosed, I enlisted into a life long research of this rare disease. I volunteered to be a guinea pig so future patients did not have to suffer through needless experimental treatments that failed. This study gave my transplant team vital information on how to treat patients like me. There are many patients that pass through the transplant process, but rarely anyone with HES (Hypereosinophilic Sydrome). This blood disorder is hard to diagnose because it mimics other diseases such as Lupus and Hodgkins.

Between infusions, a visit from Dr. Wingard, the hematologist and nutritionist consumes most of my day.

"This chair alright?" Philip asks, pointing to a recliner next to a curtainless window. I nod and sit down. The early morning sun streaks through the venetian blinds and warms the leather recliner. I reach up and scratch my bald head through a new baseball cap given to me from my kids. As I nervously scan the room, guarded about the situation, I am invisibly fastened down.

"Help yourself to a drink in the fridge if you want one. It's safe to take your mask off in here," said a nurse.

I glance up, the bill of the hat shadowing my face. She wore a scrub the color of green apples. It occurrs to me that I compared most things to food; I guess because I missed the taste of it. I couldn't help myself. The outfit is perfect for her. I sit stiff in the chair with unacknowledged fear, not daring to speak. I am a shy person by nature and in this room full of people, I feel oddly alone. Some are watching TV while reading, others are playing cards or board games with their caregiver. Some stretched and wiggled a bit, then settled back to sleep. Within a few days though, I opened up and made friends. I realized that we're all in the same boat, so it is comforting to relate to someone that is living it too.

Luckily this day only brings a unit of magnesium, so a bag is connected and the fluid is started. It is warm going in and it gives a metal taste in my mouth.

I hear a voice beside me,

"It's not as bad as you think."

I look over at this stranger that is pale, obviously wounded from his fight to live. At first I didn't say anything, but looking down at my hands I speak,

"Thank you. I need to hear that,"

He leans over to me and says, "maybe this is a sign."

"A sign? There's no such things as signs."

He leans closer, "I'm old and really shouldn't be here. I was sent to you. My name is Don Reuman. Will you be my friend?" He whispers.

After a moment I grin and nod. I see this frail man wearing a dark blue toboggan and black jogging suit, although I couldn't imagine him running anywhere. And an uncanny sense of humor bubbling to the surface. He seems well educated, but also widely self-taught. His mannerism has a distinctive style and his words flowed with meaning. He is one of those people that you meet and feel like you've known them always. It seems his life is missing something and I would help him find it. I already liked this easy going, lovable person. His wife smiled at him as if it is his nature. She put her cross stitch down to introduce herself. Jackie is a petite lady who has aged gracefully, which makes her younger looking than her spouse. There is visible signs of a life irrevocably altered; this changed who she is and who she will be. Profoundly thrust into the caregiver role in an ocean of time, she and Philip share a common role. Her compassion and love for Don is obvious. His career spent traveling the vast seas in the Navy gives him a worn leathery appearance. They compliment each other and seem to belong together, like Matt Dillon and Kitty from that old western television show.

Days turn into weeks as I struggle for a sense of normalcy; a sense of worth. My children are allowed to visit now that I'm in transplant housing. I am very weak and my appetite less desired, I still manage to enjoy my family. Someone stays with me around the clock to make sure I eat, take medications on time, and keep my appointments. My family rotates a week at a time, so Philip can return to work. I don't venture outside much. I'm to afraid of germs. I find some solace in my love of art. Katie and Haley help me design and paint a ceiling tile to hang in the hospital. Everyone touched by a transplant are given the opportunity to do a tile, supplies included. There are some done by family members in memory of a patient that lost the fight, but a majority of the art work are from survivors.

When I have an extremely exhausting day, I yearn for my mother. I miss her not here when I need her, I miss the smell of her lotion, her touch, her encouraging stories. The trauma of her death illuminates a scene in my memory of the night she died, the casket, the funeral, and the burial next to my brothers. I remember going to buy the casket with my brother. I didn't realize there were so many different styles. Dale and I walked around for over an hour, looking for the one that most resembled my mother. After all, this was her tomb. I chose a soft coral casket with a white bed of roses and a real mattress and pillow. I modeled the outfit she would wear, careful to choose one that hid the bruises. How impressed I was with the gorgeous flowers that draped the room at the funeral home. At the grave site, sitting numb next to my brother, his arm around me as if to say, "I'm her for you sis." Afterwards, I couldn't bring myself to leave. I watched as they lowered the casket; I thought it would never stop. I wondered how deep did they dig? I slowly walked over and looked in. The hole seemed so big, I wanted to leap in. I couldn't stand the thought of leaving my mother there, I wanted her back. I needed her so badly. It wasn't fair she left me to deal with life without her. With Dale at my side we grieved our loss. I stood there sobbing, looking at my mother and my brothers graves.

"We're orphans, Dale, orphans!" I still see it like it was yesterday.

I grow tired of the endless bouts of vomiting and diarrhea that racks my body. The transplant unit has three bedrooms and a full size kitchen. I stay in the master bedroom on one end; I spend a lot of time there. My caregiver scrubs and disinfects everything constantly to eliminate any type of contamination. My family worries that I might fall into depression again, and encourage me to get out and go for short walks or join them in the living room.

Philip finds me bent over the toilet and reaches for a washcloth to wipe my face. Throwing up seemed to be the normal thing to do.

"Look, I think I see an organ in there," I joke.

"Supper's ready,"

"I'll be along shortly, after I catch my breath. You go ahead."

"I'm sorry. Do you want me to do anything?" he ask, wiping my face and neck with the cool damp cloth. "Are you gonna make it?"

"Yeah, no big deal." I groan.

A journal is kept to monitor my intake, and outgoing (whichever end), and weight. It's a roller coaster with my weight. I hover in the middle nineties to one hundred pound range. I have no appetite because everything taste like cardboard. At this point, it doesn't matter because I vomit shortly after a meal anyway. It seems the only thing I can handle is clear soup or a plain baked potato.

All bone marrow transplant patients, have side effects from the transplant called GVHD (graft-versus-host disease). GVHD occurs when the donors immune cells (T-cells) don't recognize the host and attacks. Inside the hosts body is a war between the donor cells and their cells. Their skin breaks out in a fiery rash. It itches like they have rolled over and over in poison ivy. To prevent damage to the skin and any infection, gloves are recommended. The use of cyclosporine and methotrexate creams provide some relief.

I am not alone in this misery. Looking around the blue room, I notice everyone is coated in cream too. We laugh and tease each other and compare the home remedies we have concocted to alleviate the symptoms. My group consists of twelve patients that went through the transplant process at the same time and a bond is formed early. We are like a family. The youngest patient is Chase who is four years old and comes to the blue room for his infusions in a red wagon that's modified into a bed filled with toys and stuffed animals. He looks so precious wrapped up in blankets and holding his teddy. It's hard to see this innocent child suffer needlessly. His mother cradles her sick little boy and sings quietly. He lies motionless while he receives his infusion. He is the baby of three boys and is her second child to fight leukemia. There is an eleven year old girl who is the size of a fourth grader. She reminds me of a tiny porcelain doll with power white skin. She stays cocooned by a curtain around her recliner, embarrassed of her looks and spells of vomiting. Although we try to make her feel apart of our "family," she's satisfied with only the company of her grandmother. I really don't remember her name, but I felt sorry for her. AJ is a warm hearted twelve year old African American boy that stayed across the hall from me. I never found out his real name; we just called him AJ. He suffers from sickle cell. The oldest bone marrow patient is Don Reuman who is sixty eight. The rest of us are various ages in between.

One patient and his wife sit catty corner from me. His limbs so thin and transparent, he looks seven feet tall. His lankiness reminds me of my brother Ray who was built like that.

I remember as a child playing in the loft of a barn with my brothers. At six years old, Ray was already careless with his body. Like all boys he wore his scares proudly. Standing at the edge, I peered out the loft.

"Get back, you're gonna fall and break your neck!" Dale scolded me.

"Fish pish. I won't break my neck Dale."

"Watch me!" Ray shouted as he sprang past us, whoosh out the opening. A second later we heard a thud. Dust bellowing out around him, he rolled over and over again trying to catch his breath. He thought the sheet tied around his neck and wrists would help him fly.

"Are you alright, Ray? Did you break your neck?" I cried.

All I heard in response were groans from under the old dust covered sheet.

"You big dummy! What's it gonna take for you to learn that you ain't no super hero?" Dale hollered down at him.

That was just the beginning of many failed dare devil attempts Ray endured.

Sitting in the blue recliner, this man looked more like a bundle of sticks. Once a mountain of a man, his emaciated frame towers over his tiny wife even in a sitting position. He constantly plays with his hat as if he bought it to big. It is obvious that his illness has been long term. He is the first to pull a bag of medicine out and soon everyone in the room follows suite. My bag consisted of Dilantin, Cefuroxime, Prograf, Mepericine/Promethazine, Dapsone, Warfarin, Copegus, Prednisone, Pot Chl, Valtrex, Phenazopyridine, Cyclosporine and Methotrexate among other home remedy lotions I've concocted for my ailments. This is pretty much the average drug list for a majority of the patients unless they're diabetic or young, and require additional medication. One day he is in his usual place in the room and the next day, his chair is empty. *Something has gone terribly wrong. I didn't even get a chance to know him very well.* Everyone soon realizes what has happened. Over time one by one patients slowly vanish, never to be seen again. The hardest pill to swallow when children succomb to cancer. A part of me feels guilty for still living. Most of the patients inter the transplant process in a delicate physical shape, and like myself it's the last chance for survival. There is no such thing as a little miracle or a big miracle. When your faced with a life threatening disease any miracle will do.

I plop down in my favorite recliner next to the window. The sun beaming in warms my nourishment deprived body. The dread of getting sick in front of anyone, I scan the room with a nervous expression on my face.

"I'll say, you'll only get some blood today," Don explains.

"Really now?" I respond in a hoarse voice.

He smiles as he reaches over and pats my hand. I like him. I feel his warmth. He has that magical aura about him that could cook up a formula to make the desert bloom. A few minutes later, he points to his IV bag, "Look, I have the same as you." He chuckles.

With a faint smile, I acknowledge him.

"You're on the last leg of this. It's a lot easier if you stay focused on the good that will come out of all this suffering. I'm old and have seen to many dear friends leave this world before they experience the great joy that comes with aging. I know I am sometimes forgetful. But there again, some of my life is just as well best forgotten. I am blessed to have lived long enough to see my children grown and have my hair turn gray. And have my laughs be forever etched on my face. As I've got older, it is easier to be positive. I care less about the things I can't change. I don't question it anymore." He pauses to see if I am listening and continues, "I overheard you say that your parents have passed away, so Jackie and I would like to adopt you it's okay?"

I am speechless and very moved by his words. *Is he serious?* Suddenly I imagined the best case father-daughter scenario. I'll have a father that will fill my needs. Instantly I feel excited that this wonderful man whom I had only known a short time wanted to be in my life. My childhood flashed back and instantly envisioned growing up with him and all the good times spent as his only daughter. Then the thought of tossing my own father out like old tattered shoes tears at me. As if to read my mind he adds,

"It's okay to have two dad's."

"I'll buy that," I agreed.

I study this slender, slightly balding, father figure with new meaning. He speaks softly as if drained from the end of another long day at work.

"I think I need to reintroduce myself," he says through smiling lips.

"My name is Don, but you can call me Daddy Don."

I clap my hat on my head as soon as I leave the blue room. I felt like yelling loud enough to scare the birds and reach the heavens.

I smile to myself, *Thank you Lord for bringing Don my way.* I'm walking with a purpose, I have found someone new to share my life with. I feel like the luckiest woman in the world. I know if it is God's will, I will have a future with my new adopted dad.

After dishing up a bowl of soup for me, Bettye sat it on a plate and put the plate in my lap.

"There now, take your time, and try to eat this."

Bettye, now there is a wonder woman. How she came forward to help with the kids and manage the family, all her personal things, and still makes time to come here for me. I'll never know. I thought as I wipe my mouth with a napkin.

"This soup is really good. It taste like homemade."

A knock on the door interrupts the conversation. Wiping her hands on a towel, Bettye opens the door.

"Hello there, come in. Have you had supper yet? We're just finishing up." She holds the door open for Don and Jackie.

"Yes we have, thank you," Jackie said.

Don walks over and sits in the chair next to me.

"I've been thinking."

I turn to look at him, still slurping the soup from the oversize spoon.

"Would you like to come over and play Dominos?" He asks.

His shinny scalp catches the lamplight and the lines in his face giving his already broad forehead more skin.

"Whatever gave you the idea I'd even consider such a thing?"

Everyone erupts in laughter. Ah, it is so easy to laugh with him.

"I don't know how to play. I've heard about the game though." I said.

"I'll teach you kido and everyone that stays with you if they want," he replies.

"You better watch out. Don hates to loose!" Jackie jokes.

"I'm not a competitive person. No use in undue stress over a game, but I'll give it a shot."

We gather around Don and Jackie's table and he begins teaching my family and I the game of Dominos. Soon we are skillful players. I laugh inside watching Don shake his head slowly while looking through narrow eyes, thinking of his next move. I smile at him, while fooling around with the tile pieces. After the game he playfully teases me about being more focused.

Housed in the unit behind mine, we spend an enormous amount of time together. I am thankful to have Don and Jackie close. He could out whistle the birds, and often I would think a bird is singing when, in reality, it's Don. We share a humble gratitude for the Lord's blessings and walk unashamed of our faith.

In many ways I do not recognize my life. I want so badly to be home, but the thought of leaving Don to just a memory scares me. *What if he is right about God sending him to me?* I smile to myself, D-a-d-d-y D-o-n. Isn't that a wonderful funky name?

The next week brings a new caregiver. She is my first cousin Jean Combs who lives in Orange Park just outside of Jacksonville Beach. Before she would come, I had to promise to give insulin shots to her once a day. Having dealt with shots already, I am confident that I can do it with no problem. Evening arrives on the first day Jean is with me. She is preparing the shot while I watch in anticipation already regretting my promise.

"Don't look so serious, it's not working," she jokes. As she pulls her shirt sleeve up, I wrinkle my nose in fear. Jean looks at me with a smile.

"What?"

"What, what?" I glance at her.

"What are you waiting for?"

Memories of the painful interferon shots flood my mind. My eyes well up with water; my hands sweaty.

"I can't do this. I'm sorry Jean. I thought I could."

"You can. You have to. I'm here now." She coaxed.

My stomach is doing flip-flops I'm so scared. Tears soak up my face. I blink rapidly to clear my vision. I hold my breath as the needle pierces her skin. In an instant it is over.

"Man, that was easy!" I laugh.

We spend every night next door playing Dominos. It to is the first time Jean has ever played. Every evening Jackie brings out some sort of dessert to offer. It's nice to share my family with my newly adoptive parents.

One day, Jean and I get a surprise visit from my cousin Arbutus Guess who lives in New Albany, Indiana. She is named after my father's sister, so everyone calls her Little Boots for short. Growing up, I didn't have a chance to visit them very often, but now as adults, we keep in touch. Every winter she and her husband Jon drive down to Florida so see family. This year's trip includes a visit to transplant housing.

With a card in hand and tears in her eyes, she offers it to me. I open the card and a check for one thousand dollars falls out.

"This couldn't have come at a better time. Thank you Bootsie."

"God has blessed Jon and I with good health and good jobs, so I want to help you and Philip. It's a gift. Not a loan. You are family and we take care of each other. I love you Lisa." She said.

We gather around for a group hug. I am so grateful for support in my time of need. She gave her love and financial help freely.

Philip arrives the next week for his turn to stay with me. Sara and Katie are in school, so he brings little Haley. I can't keep my hands off of her. I have missed her dearly. She has changed so much since I had been away. I cherish every minute I have with her. Philip gives me a Domino set of my own. Haley and I play a modified version of Dominos. Still very weak, I don't have the strength to wrestle around with her or stay outside very long. *She is so innocent, so impressionable. I'm afraid that she'll get use to me being gone.*

On the third day of Haley's visit, I wake with painful stomach cramps. I struggle to make it to the bathroom before I collapse on the floor. I have never, ever experienced pain like this. I am drenched in a cold sweat and vomit uncontrollably. "Jesus, its getting worse!" I cry.

Philip holds my head up while he calls the ambulance. He had hoped that I was past all this rejection process, but my body is still in turmoil.

In the emergency room a tube is fed up my nose and into my stomach. Charcoal is pumped down, but as soon as it hits the stomach I vomit. The process is repeated again and again I vomit. Philip calls the BMT ward and the emergency room is instructed to send me up to the ward immediately. I am diagnosed with a severe case of gastroenteritis and admitted. I am on a morphine drip to dull the pain. It saddens me to have missed this precious time with my child. The person she relies on the most has left her again. I lay in bed and stare out my room. At night the hallways are illuminated by individual white beams, each one glowing until midnight, when the main lights are unceremoniously snapped off leaving the hall and nurse's station dimly lit. Sleep slowly engulfs me and with it brings nightmares.

I was eight years old and helping mama set the table. This meal had been served more than thirty years ago, but I still felt as though I could smell the individual flavors. I see her at the stove, whisking flour into a pan letting it swirl and dissolve. Her pale skin and eyes and delicate features complete my vision. As she wipes her hands on her apron, she pivots to get some milk out of the fridge. She is preoccupied by her cooking, which was constant and difficult. The tip of the apron licks the gas flame on the stove top and suddenly her cotton apron is engulfed in flames. She screams for help as the intense heat radiates from her body. She is burned alive.

I spring up in bed soaked in a cold sweat, gasping for air. *How could this be? My mother died of breast cancer. Is she trying to tell me something? Maybe that my life here on earth will end in a horrible, painful death.*

Philip stays for an additional week to give me extra time with Haley. I can't believe it's Easter already. We hunt eggs on the lawn in front of my transplant unit. Philip walks Haley around the perimeter of the yard while she fills her basket with candy filled eggs. Daddy Don and Mama Jackie join us for the afternoon of family fun. It concerns me that Don doesn't wear a mask when he's outside. I know it's uncomfortable and hard to breath through, but it's the way it's got to be for now. I'm terrified of germs and if the doctor says to wear a mask, I do. I also purchased two portable air filters for my unit; one in my room and one in the living room. As the day blends into the evening we all enjoy some of Jackie's homemade peach cobbler. The aroma of the cobbler transports me once again back to my childhood: I was in the kitchen helping my mother peel peaches—clear as day.

The sun slowly ends its journey over the horizon, casting oblique shades of orange and gray. I want to curl up and sleep. I slip inside the bed. It's cold in there, like a pond. The room is hushed and shadowed. Philip kisses the hollow of my cheek.

"I love you, you know that."

"I love you, too." I whisper.

"We'll always belong together," he says.

I know there is a implicit second half to his sentence, that maybe he means: "We'll always belong together even when you're gone."

One of the best ways to fend off unwanted negative thoughts for me is prayer. I pray for God, the angels and spirit guides to protect me. Over the course of several years living with cancer, I have learned to forgive myself for everything.

9

I worry about Don. He looks fragile and ruined: the transplant process has changed him, so much that I barely have memories of our first encounter. I remember the gleam in his eyes, the feel of his hand resting gently on the top of my bald head. To me he is the most caring man in the world.

Then one unusually beautiful day the long-dreaded occurred. Peering over my mask I see Jackie standing in the hallway outside the lab. Her brown eyes look tired and heavy.

"When you get done with your labs, meet me in the blue room, okay?" she said.

I swallow hard to pass by the lump in my throat. I am speechless. All I do is nod.

My mind is racing. *What's wrong with my daddy Don? Lord please let him be alright.*

I stand in the doorway of the exam room. I feel something twist slightly inside me with sudden panic threatening to overtake me. Daddy Don is looking down at the luminous dial of his wristwatch. I know this is one of those abysmal times when despair visits men, when insomniacs writhe in an ocean of silence, when the jobless and the bankrupt want to scream in order to break their risks of the course of action, when solders abruptly awake to the beginning of coming battle. He seems composed and speaks with passable courage and calm. Without looking up he says to me,

"Lisa, honey, I've got some bad news and I want to talk to you first before I give my answer to Dr. Wingard."

The overhead light in the room illuminates the oval of his face. I study it and in many ways I did not recognize him. I wonder what he has to tell me and secretly hoping for the best. This tall, gentle, and thoughtful man has become a del facto father in my life and I thank God for him. I walk over to him and look up into his sky blue eyes which now appear dark. I can feel something is very wrong. I don't know what it is, but I know it was something. Well, actually deep down I did know, but I chose not to face it, maybe hide it from myself somehow. I don't like to see him like this. It is frightening to say the least.

"What's wrong daddy Don?"

He inhales deeply and begins, determined to charm away the sulk, his philosophy of handling ups and downs.

"I have a decision to make and I want you to help me make it. Whatever you say, I'll go with it."

"What do you mean?" I ask grudgingly.

I see his spirit unsatisfied, rapidly exhausting the instinct to live. He sighed, inhaled as if to speak, then appeared to rethink himself. Finally, in a hoarse whisper, I said,

"I suppose you are going to tell me what I don't want to hear."

"Well," he paused again as to carefully pick the right words.

"The transplant has failed, but they still have enough of the donor cells left if I want to try it again. What do you want me to do?"

My tear ducts releases a flow like a raging river on its journey to the ocean. He wraps his arms around me and holds me tight to his chest. I hear the sound of his heart thudding. I hear it clearly through his chest wall. The warm, solid feel of his arms gives me a sense of protection. My eyes fill with unashamed and unstoppable tears. I pull away and look up at him, those blue eyes smiling down at me.

"But, are you strong enough?"

"If I start right away, then yes."

A wave of emotions engulfed my soul. I am tempted to rail against him, to demand to know who he thought he was to admit that he had worthless faith. *I'll completely fall apart if I lose another father,* raced through my mind.

"Of course the answer is yes! You once told me, on these very grounds that you would do anything I ask, even to the ultimate degree."

"They're gonna be obstacles, and there's no guarantee."

"Daddy Don, you've faced obstacles coming into this transplant already, so what's the difference this time. I'm only interested in the outcome."

He gently wipes my tear soaked face. "I'll do my best."

"Your best is all I ask."

He takes my hand, poised and ready to continue the fight. Lord, keep him safe I whisper, then dry my eyes again; treasuring the way his smile creased his cheeks, and eyes that match the sky above, a Kentucky sky of a blue that deepens the more you look into it.

The rest of the day I go through the motions like every day before. Not allowing myself to think about anything, anything at all.

Kneeling at my bedside I end my prayer, "Lord, please help me to understand this. Help me to have patience, to look to you for comfort. This is so hard for me."

I lay in bed wondering if I have ask too much of Don. At sixty-eight, he is the oldest transplant patient and a risky task to accomplish a second time. His unrelated donor was found in the northern United States and once notified that he was a match for Don, he unselfishly donated the marrow. This is a procedure is the same as a biopsy involving the extraction of bone marrow from the hip. Don is only told that the donor is in his twenties and if the transplant is successful, at the donor's permission, the recipient is allowed to contact them. There are countless survival stories from this simple gift of life. Until my illness, I did not realize how extensive the bone marrow donor network of people were involved in this life saving organization.

That night my dreams are filled with memories of my own father. I was about five years old looking up from my coloring book to see this tired, coal miner walking across the laquer covered wood floor of the living room. As he passed by, the wood creaking at the weight of each step. He had a look of despair as though seized by dour mood as if he saw his hopes, his self worth vanishing. I thought he could be a better man. I wanted a better life for him. His clothes were always covered in coal dust. What was he but dirty? Dirty of his body, dirty of his spirit. How he looked in the picture on the fireplace mantel in his army uniform taken before I was born. That was the handsomest uniform I ever had seen-though at my age, I hadn't seen any other. Later at the supper table, I watched him over the rim of my glass of milk as he devoured his food. I followed him as he walked outside in the late evening to gather eggs for breakfast. Small flocks of chickens were noisily attacking the ground. "Better run before daddy catches you!" I hollered at the yard birds. I watched my father and brothers pound nails into the loose fence gate that kept the plowing mule corralled in the old broken-down barn. He and my brothers work furiously before the daylight ebbed away.

Winter mornings in North Florida are rarely harsh, and this morning is sweeter than usual. A week-long warming trend has fooled the crape myrtle trees into early bloom. From the window I watch Philip stretch and pelt across the lawn to the sidewalk. Jogging has always been his avenue for stress release. It is a deliciously brisk morning with the air fresh and clean, having been washed by a torrential nighttime downpour. He starts jogging, pacing himself so he doesn't run out of steam. Thirty minutes later, he ends back at transplant housing, straddle legged and bent over to catch his breath, chest pumping like his legs.

"This feels good, I need to run more often. In high school it was no big deal for me to run twenty miles just for pleasure," he says between sucks of air. I envision him tall and lean running with long easy strides through the country outside of Bainbridge, tennis shoes slamming into the ground. Traci ran with him on her visits to Shands. They would run from transplant housing down to the hospital and back. At five feet eight she had no problem keeping pace with him.

I don't always address my problems how he deals with his, but not dealing with things that can make a difference will only fester. When my emotions overwhelm my thoughts, I feel like a woman carrying a lamp in the night. I try to ignore the problem in the hope that somehow it will work itself out. In fact I'm only setting myself up for failure.

A week later, Don is back on the bone marrow ward preparing for his second transplant.

"I love you, daddy Don."

I know you do. This will turn out for the best. I'm sure; you wait and see. I can't begin to tell you how much you mean to me." He says through dry pale lips.

We spend as much time together before he is back behind a plexiglass wall.

Looking at the world outside the window of my temporary home. I glance to the west to catch lightning fracturing the sky.

"A storm's coming." Philip says as he sits down next to me.

"I know. I can smell it. We sure need rain, but I'm for a slow gentle two-day steady fall instead of a downpour." I said.

Thunder rolls far off, the dry ground screaming for a drink. Lightning came closer this time, and the thunder answering a few seconds later. The storm moves near, and soon I am lost in thought. My mind's ripe with visions of Don. He has the ability to make me smile when nobody else can. "If corn oil is made from corn, and vegetable oil is made from vegetables, then what is baby oil made from?" He jokingly asks me. I burst out laughing at his silly questions. He entertained me with stories of the war and places he was stationed. How he graduated from high school and graduated into the military world almost the same day. How he served what seemed a lifetime on a gun ship in the Navy and spent time in the Orient among other places.

I don't believe I overstate when I say I know of no man, who was more universally loved and respected. He loved his country with all his heart and soul. There were many men in public life who at times made a more brilliant showing than Don; there were others who seemed better fashioned who dazzled and filled the public eye, but he was just one of many that served in the shadows. If not for the men behind the scenes, banding together there wouldn't be a military. As I listened to his extraordinary tales of his adventures, I realized he had a great, unselfish, human heart; a heart full of kindness, even toward those that despitefully used him.

He talked about his big farm house on a several acres of land in a small town near Ocala, Florida. I formed a mental image of working next to him feeding the ducks, chickens, collecting eggs, and putting the horses out to pasture. I wish that our paths had crossed years earlier. Oddly I feel cheated.

I love his admirable qualities, excellent common sense; a man who has shown me things that are not learned from books or taught in schools, but from experience. He came from poverty and through adversity he came, working his way upward with both his heart and simple unbroken ascent to a higher place. And now I see him again struggling and suffering.

I pray for final and deserved success.

I spend as much time with Don as allowed. So much in life seems to be a struggle; it makes me wonder why I am here. In this unfortunate process, there is no shortcut. The suffering is long and thoughts of despair crowd my mind. Is this the right decision? Did I hurt myself and others in the process? I believe there is a God and I believe our difficult challenges in life are really blessings in disguise. He won't give us more than we can handle. I'm not afraid of life after death, I'm afraid of the process of dying.

Standing in the doorway I speak through a mask,

"I'm glad to see you looking better today."

"Lisa! Come sit down," Don pats the bed next to him. "I had a dream last night and I want to tell you all about it."

Jackie waves me in and I make myself comfortable. His room feels warm and cozy with lamps and scented candles about. Jackie gave it her special touch to make it feel more like a bedroom instead of a hospital room. It is obvious she gives overflowing cups of love to Don.

"I don't know if it was a dream or for real. I want to say it wasn't a dream. I was asleep and someone was calling out my name. I opened my eyes and sat up in bed. At first I thought it was Jackie, but she wasn't in here. I looked over to the door and I saw an angel dressed in a white gown. A bright glow illuminated from all around her, and at her feet lay a newborn baby girl. The angel said, "this is your child." Before my eyes I watched the baby grow into a child, then a teenager, and to an adult. I couldn't believe what I saw before me. I recognized her deep blue eyes, the dimple in her chin, her gorgeous smile. Lisa, it was you! I never told you that I lost my only daughter. She was stillborn on December 3rd, 1960."

The hair on my arms stood up! With tears in my eyes,

"Daddy Don, that's my birthday."

Don gave a hearty laugh, "See, I knew you belonged to me. You look just like my boys."

I didn't know what to say. I thought that he wanted me to be his child so bad that it had consumed him.

I embraced the idea of him as my father. My own father deserted me which cheated me out of a father-daughter relationship. My younger siblings ask fewer questions about the abandonment, but I was forced to accept the loss in stages, slowly closing one door and moving on the next. I didn't have a chance to be a daddy's girl: he didn't give me a chance to love him. I had empty spaces in my life; a gaping hole that sits permanently in my soul. I guess this is why I try to soak up as much of Don's love as I can, a quickly as possible, as if excess today will guarantee a tomorrow. He filled that empty space, to father me, to awaken feelings I lost or possibly never had.

Don came into my life at precisely the right time, so much so that I was convinced that I didn't need the one thing I didn't have. With him in my life I am able to rid myself of all the built up denial, anger, betrayal and lack of acceptance. His love allowed me to face my grief that I had locked up in a sealed file somewhere in my soul and reawakened my need for a father.

Don is progressing wonderfully. He's gaining strength and his spirits are high.

"When I get out of here and back in transplant housing, I want us to take a trip down to the coast and do some site seeing; we'll have a splendid time. I know a nice little place to eat that over looks the bay. Your cousin Jean is welcome to come too," he said.

"But daddy Don, we're not suppose to leave the area. I'm scared for you because you won't wear a mask. As long as you promise to wear a mask and tell me when your tired then I'll go."

"Okay, Lisa Ann," he jokes.

It is another three weeks before he is well enough to take our trip. It is an unfavorable opinion of the transplant ward to leave the area, but the need to get away from the constant struggles is worth it. We act like little children doing something that will get us in trouble, but the first sight of the picturesque coast makes it worthwhile.

It is early afternoon when we all troop up the stairs that has no banister. Obviously week from lack of exercise, I order my thundering heart to slow down as I take deep breaths. Once we are all seated with menus in hand, I feel alive and free. *How long has it been since we'd laughed and joked like this? Months? Weeks, even?* I wondered. I realize that this is only temporary, it nonetheless stokes a small flame of hope for brighter days. I notice that Don is eyeing me curiously, almost forcing himself in my thoughts.

Don asks, "anyone for desert?" We all shake our heads, Don waves for the waitress.

After lunch, we walk around the square window shopping and enjoying the scenery. It's a friendly place, a small seaside community where, if you stopped three or four people on the street, at least one of them would know the whereabouts of the person you were looking for or at least the family.

The Bible says, "I am to live in the day, this day, not years before or years hence." I am living this day, and enjoying every minute of it. Soon it will end and so will my time with Don. He's improving everyday and like it or not, I will have to simply surrender to my life here without him. As the trees in the autumn let go of their leaves, so does the time come to let Don go. I see it happen and suddenly, it seems, the woods are bare.

No words can express the happiness in my heart that Don is on his way to recovery, so much that he is released from Shands and transplant housing. Recovery means different things to different people, but to me it means I carry on this fight without my father-figure, my mentor, my gift from God. In my minds eye, I am losing more than a companion, I am losing a part of me. The heaviness and fear that he will forget me engulfed my heart completely. He exposed my heart to a more peaceful vision of love. Now I can release all the anger towards my father; there was so much of it that I just didn't know how to cope with it. I was always afraid of my father. He could always say something mean to make me cry, and it tore my heart out. I was the daughter of a distant father, who had little involvement in my life and I withdrew emotionally. I was very resentful about him leaving me. Don broke that wall down and I allowed myself to greave my father's death. I finally understood his demeanor was the result of addiction to alcohol which emphasized his inability to take on the expressive parenting role. Don was instrumental in getting my father and me on a higher level and patch up what had eroded my soul. I now have forgiven my father for being a very angry man.

Our last day together is a mixture of joy and sadness all swirled around in my heart. I know that Don fiercely loves me and that he would willingly hand over his own life to ensure I have the best of one. Subconsciously I want so bad for him to stay, but I put on a brave front and outwardly express excitement for him.

Before he leaves, he hands me a wrapped gift. The card is addressed to Lisa Ann. For some reason he likes using my first and middle name in conjunction.

"This is something for you, to help you cope and regain your life back."

Inside the masculine print wrapping paper, there is a five by seven picture of Don standing next to a railroad crossing sign. He's dressed in white slacks and wearing a white hat. He looked sophisticated and confident about himself, so in control—and to think that I saw him on the street, he'd be the one of those men I'd admire, one that I would be certain holds the knowledge that so many others lack. Under the picture, is a plaque with the inscription of the Jabez prayer. He leans over and reads it to me.

"Jabez cried out to the God of Israel, "Oh that you would bless me indeed, and enlarge my territory, that your hand would be with me, and that you would keep me from evil, that I may not cause pain!" So God granted him what he requested, 1 Chronicles 4:10. Lisa, I want you to put this somewhere visible and read it so often that you memorize it. God listens to our prayers and if it's his will, he will grant your request."

Standing on weak knees, I watch them drive away, Don in the passenger seat waving and blowing kisses. Tears soaking up my face, I return the motions of goodbye. Philip holds me steady with his hand over mine, squeezing tight. The last vision I have of him is his open hand pressed against the window as if to say, "I'll always be with you."

10

I gaze with fixed eyes at Don's vacant unit behind me. The rain pouring like open vessel of water making a misty haze rising up from the ground. The wind howling through the trees only intensifies the emptiness. A blanket around my shoulders and over my head, my mind ripe with visions of months, weeks, days spent with the most precious people I know. Lost in thought, the tears oozing through the corners of my eyes. I relive his every joke, his every laugh, and his encouraging words that somehow helped me manage to forget all the suffering and put me in a better place. Sometimes my memory plays tricks on me, but this memory I'll keep alive for the rest of my life. Don and Philip have so much in common; through them I have realized that I am who I am and that makes me unlike anyone else. I have a right to be different, not constantly hiding imperfection or signs of weakness. They taught me to look at the big picture, to see how far I have come from where I was, and that getting by just gets me by, but taking chances and walking that extra step will get me anywhere I want to go. A place before cancer invaded my life.

I concentrate on my desire of full recovery and to be set free from the burdens of post transplant. My busy schedule did not allow time to brood over the previous day's events, nor did it give me time to worry. By the end of the day, I am physically and mentally exhausted.

Before long Don's unit is occupied by another transplant family. I watch Philip help the couple unload their luggage and other items from the trunk. It's obvious that the man is the transplant patient with his face concealed by a mask. He sits motionless in a lawn chair Don had left behind. The sun warming his thin frame covered by jeans that once fit and a jersey that consumes his torso. His toddler running in circles arms stretched out for wings making airplane sounds.

"Do you want to go over tomorrow and met our new neighbors?" Philip ask.

"Yeah, I guess so."

He said nothing more, instead gives me the space I need to gather myself.

A new day brings a phone call from Don. We discuss my blood counts, what infusions I had, and my progress. I hear enthusiastic agreement in his voice, but I feel an underlying expression of sorrow for leaving me behind. I assure him that I'm still working toward my goal of complete recovery. He ends the call saying,

"Surely this short time apart isn't going to make a difference in all the years we will have together."

My mind takes off on another daydream—Don's smiling face as he shows off his country village he constructed for his trains. The model consumes the two car garage with fine gravel, realistic cottages, stores, farm houses complete with livestock shadowed by mountains and trees. His feet refusing to stand still, as he paces willing the trains through the tunnels and over the countryside.

Oh daddy Don, how I miss you. I almost chuckle. We talk and joke for what seems hours. I am sad one minute, overjoyed the next.

April 27, 2003, I am on the down hill slide to the one hundred day limit. Surprisedly I still suffer from stomach problems, graph verses host and weight loss. I hover around ninety five pounds, I have no appetite (everything taste like cardboard)—I look anorexic. I look in the mirror and I realize how haggard I am beginning to look. At forty one years old, I look sixty. My complexion shallow with dark circles under my eyes. For the most part, I tolerate vanilla or strawberry nutritional drinks, Jell-O or clear soup over solid food. My immediate impulse is to tell Don, but I know that it will only intensify his worries about me, so I continue to force myself to eat light amounts of solids to keep my strength up.

"I don't want you to starve." Philip holds out a container.

It's a plain baked potato from the restaurant down the street.

"Leave it to you, Philip, to go beyond what I ask for." I joke. "I don't know what I would do without you."

"You don't have to worry about chief Philip going anywhere," he says with a chuckle.

I sit on the front stoop and nibble at my potato while watching white clouds that fluff against the sky like fresh feathers. Something I see everyday, but now just in a different way.

Elton and Bettye leave Valdosta and Traci to oversee the household until Philip comes home. It's their time to exchange caregiver duties with Philip. Sometimes a catastrophic illness wrecks more homes than national disasters, and the thought of being away from my children manifested itself as a deep ache in the center of my chest. The thought drains all my strength and I blamed everything, but I blamed myself most of all, for my illness.

The sixty first day of post transplant begins as usual. I do the morning ritual of labs and then waiting in the blue room for the results. This morning I am called back to the lab for additional blood to be drawn.

"What's this? You going to leave me any?" I joke.

The technician smiles and hands the tubes to his assistant. I sit in silence searching for any clues of something abnormal.

A memory of my mother floods my mind. Her long slender legs walked the length of the enormous porch as she scanned the yard for any of her children. Too many shrubs and bushes to see through, so she walked slowly down the concrete steps and into the yard. My brother and I concealed ourselves like panthers in wait, stalking our prey. In bare feet she moved in the cool moist grass of the yard, pausing at every shadow and poking every shrub with a stick. She played our game and pretended not to see us, and jumped in surprise when we sprung out to scare her.

I am lead down the hall to a private room. I am oblivious to anything around me. Dr. Wingard reaches out his hand; his handshake signifies a positive energy, but I know that he is a medical professional and right now I feel this is leading to a horrific situation. What ever he has to say, I need to muster up the courage to fight with all my might, all my soul, all my being.

"How is your day?" The doctor asks.

I look down toward the floor as if embarrassed. I smile weakly. "Fine," I said, adding "I think."

"Seems like something has happened today." my brow wrinkles as I try to explain what has happened.

"We are profoundly sorry," said the doctor.

"Doctor", I whispered, tightening the grip on the chair, "What is it? Is it bad? How bad"

He doesn't answer right away. He writes some notes on the chart.

"We did everything within our power to heal you."

I see torment on the doctor's face as he presents the lab results. I remember feeling profound sadness as Dr. Wingard explains that the leukemia has returned and it is very aggressive. My body is too weak to attempt another transplant, there's nothing else he can do for me. I can go home. That's it. That's all I remember.

Once again my life hangs in the balance. *I'm going to wake up in a minute, this is not happening. When my children needed me I was there to help; when my husband needed me I was there to help, but I can't help myself.* Where do I start facing something like this rationally. Nothing in my life has prepared me to face death when its looking straight at me—Nothing did. Nothing could. Nothing ever does. I had decided that God has forgotten me. I am stunned. And, finally, terribly frightened. I am angry—frightfully angry. I rock back and forth. How I have suffered. How I have suffered. Over and over in my mind. Why, why, why . . .

I winced.

"How is this possible?" I ask quietly.

I look past him at the dust specks, thick and heavy floating in the sunlight split into thin lines of the venetian blinds. My mind wonders. What time is it? What will we have for supper tonight?

I breath a heavy sigh and force myself to my feet. My knees are shaky; my hands trembling. I didn't know what to do. I feel trapped! *Lord help me. Give me a sign that this is just another test. He's talking like I'm already dead. It can't be over. I'm not done yet.* I tell myself to calm down and figure something out with logic and reason. I'm not dead yet. Not yet. It is my *intention* to stay positive. After everything I've been through, the chemo, experimental drugs, losing my hair—twice, I have simply decided that I am no good to anyone if I didn't try to put forward a faithful demeanor. The fact of the matter is that in the debts of my soul I am terrified and morose over this. Time is after all, all I have.

Philip breaks the bad news to our children. They are stunned and terribly frightened.

"Is she going to die daddy?" Sara asks.

"No," Philip said honestly. "She is not and don't even think it." He held onto his belief, never losing his composure. "We have to hold on to our faith that she will pull through this," he adds.

Philip arrives without remembering the trip, like he is in a deep anesthetic fog.

His first words are, "where's my baby?"

I crumble in his arms.

"How can this be happening. Everything is a blur, nothing makes any sense. I don't know what else to do. I am so tired of feeling helpless. I am tired in my mind. I am tired in my body. I close my eyes and the images of my children haunts my thoughts. If I don't make it, will they forgive me for leaving them? They say I'm dying. I can't keep holding on, I'm slipping away. I don't know why all this is happening; if I belong here or not. I'm afraid they are right that my time is up.

Holding me in his arms Philip consoles me.

"If you're dying, then I'd feel it. You've got a lot of life left in you. Don't give up, you can't give up. Your time is not up. It's not finished. I look in your eyes and through the haze I see that your faith has never diminished. I'll make this right again, with God's help, I will."

Opposites attract. That is what people say about Philip and myself. I am average, fair, talkative, while he is the quiet type, tall and handsome. A balanced relationship, warm and caring.

"I am thankful, really I am, but I sometimes feel that I'm being punished for something. Last night I prayed for God to just give me tomorrow and if it's his will for me to live long enough for Haley to remember me. I made a promise that I will teach her everything I know about Jesus and make sure our kids stay in church."

"Tomorrow will come, Lisa. We will live each day as it comes to us, whether it's pain or joy, as it is a gift. God has been good to us, he's not punishing you for anything. You've got to remember that God is always way ahead of everyone else, only he knows when you leave this earth. He's going to take care of us just wait and see."

Us—what a wonderful word. Us—as in Philip and me. I hug the thought.

"Do you want me to fix us something to drink?" he asks.

There it is again, the magic word—us. My heart turns over with love for him.

I am going home, surrounded by my things, where my children are waiting like flowers in the yard for a spring shower to call them to bloom. A part of me will always remain in Gainesville. Oddly, I only remember bits and pieces of my time here, from that wintery February day when I arrived to my unwanted departure. A spirit brave and true, I fought away the pewter clouds dripping with crystal rain. Each drop magnifies an opal rainbow without beginning or end. I don't fear death. I refuse to talk about it. I know where my soul is going when they lay me to rest. Philip is my soulmate and to death do us part, but for all worth having cannot be touched, only felt and forever cherished.

Philip and I drive back to Valdosta with only a comment every now and then. His warm calloused hand engulfs mine; his thumb making a swirling pattern softly caressing the back of my hand. My mind drifting,

I ponder how strange it was that, after such a short time, I still sometimes have difficulty grasping how much Philip and I belong to each other. How much harder it must be, then, for me, who had always been so solitary, to deal with the intensity of our feelings for each other. Yet even so, there is no part of me that he did not know, no nook or cranny of my mind into which I had not delved—though some memory, dark and painful, that to me were best left undisturbed. The love we share frightens me sometimes, even though is warms my soul. I know that our destiny is predetermined and sometimes, what life gives, it can also take back, cruelly and, more often than not, without warning. Still I could not have it any other way. My husband is the only man for me, as I am the only woman for him; for I am certain that if I had to do it again, I would choose him above all others. He alone has breached the high walls surrounding my heart and made a place for himself there, safe, secure. Only death would separate us now.

There is nothing on earth quite like a clear bright cloudless sky above me and the sound of children playing. We drive up to our home erected just a few years earlier, the house is a good one, high and, reassuringly solid; for it was framed with heavy timber and sided with hardy board. The house had been built with love and pride by my husband, its walls and floors painted as I specified. Still, much as I loved my home, I was not ready to return to it just yet. You can't always get what you want.

"I love you," Philip murmured.

Because of the kind of man he is, those words came easily to him. His low husky voice still faintly accented by his country upbringing.

"I love you, too, Philip . . . . my Philip," I sigh. "God, how I love you!"

As though to show me how much, with one hand, he tilts my face up to his and kisses me gently, very gently.

As grasshoppers spring up to avoid the chase of a lawnmower, my children swarm me. Now, on this late, summer afternoon, too thin, too pale, encumbered by the transplant and looking far older than my age, I stand outside my house and soak up all that remains of my world and dreams. And from that moment on, I have given up my battle against cancer. I totally surrender and let go of everything and let God take over.

I ease myself down on the couch and soak up my children. "I'm cooking something special for you mama," Traci says.

I manage a weak smile.

"I know. I can smell it." The aroma of peach cobbler transports me once again back to my childhood: I was in the kitchen helping my mother peel peaches to bake—clear as day.

The house looks good; secondhand furniture and all. It looks fancy to me. No one would take it for secondhand stuff. My tropical plants are thriving. Bettye has taken excellent care of them in my absence. I know every corner, every panel, every nail that I watched Philip hammer to build this house. We had rented for years. We saved and saved until we had the money for a substantial down payment. It had been strictly my idea, I didn't mind the long hours spent working side by side with Philip to save as much money possible, raising five kids, running a house, and being a postal manager.

Yeah . . . . it is good to be home.

I stand up weakly and make my way to the kitchen, where Bettye is standing over a pot. She puts the spoon down to cup my face in her thin, white hands.

"Don't cry. God's with you."

I wasn't crying, but she knew I was crying inside. With leukemia, I had a time bomb inside me, and obviously it had gone off. To my doctors, all the drugs are doing is giving me some time. This illness has taught me humility, surrender, and faith. I have to trust God and let my mind and emotions sit this one out.

I sleep till noon then get up and feel like I need a nap.

"Hey sleepy head. Are ya gonna dream the day away."

Philip is standing in the doorway, a look of amused concern on his face. Though in Philip's mind, concern and amusement are mutually exclusive terms. Philip seems to be able to combine them masterfully.

"Yeah, I feel like I just finished a marathon, I'm so weak."

With long strides, Philip walks over and sits a tray down on the night stand. He is a very handsome man, but he wears an expression of tired sadness I can't bear. I feel a tear roll down my cheek as I watch him.

I must stay strong, I can't let him down again, I tell myself.

With no appetite and feeling nauseated, I take small bites of the sandwich.

The days flow by like a calm river slowly finding it's way to the ocean. I focus on one day at a time. I see the world now in high definition. The grass looks greener, the sky is deeper, and the flowers more brilliant. Before all this, I barely had time to relax and soak in all that heaven offers; the birds singing, the sound of the wind, bumble bees dancing on the peddles of flowers or the smell of gardenia bushes that frame the house. I am for the first time enjoying life. Now I spend more time on the patio absorbing the warm sunshine. I follow Haley driving her battery operated Jeep around the perimeter of the yard while Philip stacks firewood at the edge of the property, sneezing in the dust. He removes his hat to wipe the sweat from his forehead, then puts it back on his head, looks up and smiles, and continues.

I'm standing on the beach watching the tide come in. I see the high water marks in the sand and know the waves are breaking close. I had watched my mother suffer and I know I am there. Sometimes death comes quickly for some but she and I are both taking the round about way. I don't fear death like I once did. I am at peace with myself and with the Lord. These past few weeks has opened my eyes to the raw, energetic power of the Lord in a way that I have never before witnessed. I recite the Jabez prayer constantly. The words sink into my mind, and my point of view has changed. Doctors judge a patients outlook by what they see in black and white, but I know there is a higher power that can manipulate the outcome.

One especially peaceful evening out of the blue a voice said, "another miracle."

Suddenly my stomach flip-flops. I was too blind to see that this is my opportunity to show the true meaning of the word "miracle." God didn't intervene just to play around and confuse me; he has a purpose. Nowadays we don't have visual miracles like when Moses turned the Nile into a river of blood or Noah and his family building an ark in a land thirsty for rain and gathering animals of every kind. We have miracles just the same, even if the task at hand seems impossible.

The next morning I wake with renewed vigor in the pattern of my past. I slip noiselessly out of bed, alert and on a mission. "Today is a bonus day!" I shout to the heavens. "All this time I have let Jesus carry me, but now I am gonna walk the rest of the way."

Philip sleepily agrees,

"what you have needed on this journey has been prepared for. Open your heart and laugh like you've never laughed before. You have changed in many ways, unveiling yourself like flowers unfolding to light. Throughout all this suffering, when the rain got heavy and your soul weak, Satan permeated your mind with negative thoughts. Like a vampire, he sucked out your will to live and filled you with worry and fear. As I have told you time and time again, your heart is pure, and let nobody live there, except Jesus and Jesus alone."

"You're right, Philip. I didn't see it that way, but yes. It will take all my strength and effort, all my faith, to climb up and over and then to a place where I belong."

Sunday morning I join my family in church. Out of habit, I dawn a hat and mask. Philip hesitates when I stop walking.

"Are you alright?"

"Yeah babe, just got to get my breath. I forget sometimes."

"Forget what?"

I lean a little more heavily on his arm. "I forget that I have to pace myself and be thankful."

Philip pats my hand, "I think we all forget to be thankful at times."

Our church family surrounds us with the warmest reception and treat me as a celebrity. I am painfully shy, but I find it easy to witness God's blessings. I want to share with those that are not aware of my circumstances. I felt the need to express how I have overcome unimaginable obstacles and fought perpetual weakness and disappointment to grow in my faith. In the Bible, Jesus touched a blind mans eyes and said, "Become what you believe."

Here is my story I shared it with my church:

"I would like to tell you about a woman that I know very well and the trails and tribulations she endured that would test her faith to the limit. During her pregnancy with her youngest daughter, she was told that there were problems with her blood. Eventually she was diagnosed with a very rare form of leukemia called hypereosoniphilia. This is cancer of the white blood cells instead of the red. She was labeled high risk and carefully guarded. The blood disorder continued to escalate out of hand and in the last trimester her baby was taken. Even though the baby was premature, she there were no sign of leukemia. Soon after the birth of her baby she started a rigorous regimen of drugs and chemotherapy to save her life. The excessive buildup of cancer cells in her brain caused a grand maul seizure and twelve mini strokes. Blind, paralyzed and speech impaired, she was given a minimum chance of survival and transported to Shands Hospital in the attempt to save her life. Miraculously she survived the ordeal, and had to endure the pain of physical therapy to relearn how to eat, write, and walk. In all, it takes one and half years to recover. As a last resort, a bone marrow transplant is recommended and a national donor search ensues to find a match. On February 26, 2003, she received her second chance of life. She is moved into post transplant housing for an additional one hundred days. On the sixty first day, she is told that the transplant failed. Too weak to attempt any further treatment, she is sent home.

Those here that don't know who I am talking about, it's me. I ask everyone here to pray for me. I feel in my heart that this miracle is not over. The Lord knows what we need before we ask it. I feel God's presence all around me and I know he's in charge. He works miracles to build faith, however practical or timely. I have learned to walk in his grace and mercy and work on keeping the right attitude. Letting my problems, anger, resentment get the better of me, only adds fuel to the fire. Each day is a gift.

Thank you.

After the church service, a lady ask. "Have you considered writing a book about your experience?" Her eyes swell with tears as she says,

"you need to witness to the world. These events of your life are extraordinary and the seeds of God's goodness and compassion are planted in your heart. Lisa, you will never be the same. People will take time to read your story and realize that even though their lives are a mess, they need to feel God is still there. This old world is so desperate to know the love and compassion of God. He has placed in you the potential to witness his kind, caring, loving spirit. You have the ability to show the world that miracles do exist today."

I mull over our conversation, and that night before undressing for bed. I lean against my dresser by the window and look into the starry sky. I am keyed up, I will have trouble sleeping; I know it. I open my heart and I talk to God. I feel the warmth of the Holy Spirit through out my body. It is good to have me back to where I belong.

The next two weeks pass without a second thought of anything negative. Surprisedly it is time for me to return to Shands. Many friendships were formed during my time there. Some were brief and some will last a life time. I am happy and feel very fortunate to have survived what I call a living hell. It is as if it were yesterday.

The elevator door opens on the fourth floor. To my left are the doors leading to the transplant ward and to the right is the lab, blue room and exam rooms. Soon I am met by the bone marrow staff who are delighted to see me. It feels odd having blood drawn from my arm. The catheter had been removed the day I left transplant housing.

"You look wonderful. How's life treating you?" A technician ask.

"Couldn't be better. I've survived yesterday and today and if God's willing I'll be here tomorrow."

"Well, you can't ask for more than that," he says through smiling lips.

We wait in the not so comfortable chairs of the waiting room to see Dr. Wingard. We are soon escorted back to a room down the hall.

Dr. Wingard points to a chair, "Come sit down."

I ease down in the chair, tucking my hands under my legs. Philip stands behind me; his hands jammed into his pockets.

"How have you been?" The doctor ask.

"Alright I guess."

I shift in my seat and slump slightly. Not comfortable I put my hands in my lap interlocking my fingers. He smiles. His smile is always so gentle that gives me a sense of his genuine concern.

"I have your lab results."

He opens the lab report he has in his lap and stares at me, his smile widening. Philip rest his hand on my shoulder. I inhale and subconsciously hold my breath. I peer into his eyes as if they are mirrors reflecting the writing on the report. My lungs ache; I realize that I am holding my breath and release the pressure on my lungs.

"The report shows your hemoglobin is 13.3, white blood cell count 4.4, platelet count 108,000 and 37.4 eosinophil. Everything looks good with the exception of your magnesium is low."

Clearing my throat and swallowing hard, "what does it mean?"

Philip sits down beside me and pulls me lose. He feels the tension knotting my limbs.

"What I'm saying is that the eosinophil count is almost ten points from when you were discharged a few weeks ago. Had I not been here to see it myself, I would not have believed it. Impressive—that is all I can say."

This is dramatic. What I am hearing, in an instant all the suffering and disappointments I had gone though is now a memory. It has come into a complete circle like an awkward stain glass mosaic, forming a jerky map that in the end transformed into a beautiful masterpiece. I cry tears of joy and pray aloud, "thank you Jesus, thank you God, thank you Dr. Wingard."

Philip stands in one smooth motion, pulling me to my feet and wraps his arms around me.

"Now this is the best news I've heard yet. Come on, we're going home."

Today I am considered by medical standards a walking miracle. I have beat the odds and I am in complete remission. I no longer take life for granted. I know from a personal perspective, I will never be the same again and I treat everyday as a gift. I understand that now, better that I ever have before. I am living proof that there is a God and he is above all. I have walked in the shadow of death and searched for pleasant places, the things that I love; my Lord, my husband, my children, and found that I am richly blessed. My dear daddy Don passed away in December, 2003. He had always wanted a daughter and loved me as his own. My mother once said, "find a blessing in everything." Someday I too will join loved ones that touched my life in Heaven and I will be forever free.

I hope that my story of a miracle will help those who are searching for a reason to carry on and will find the strength and renewed faith that there is a higher power in charge.